VAGUS NERVE SELF STIMULATION

THE BEGINNER'S GUIDE TO MANAGE ANXIETY, STRESS, DEPRESSION AND LIVE A HEALTHY LIFE

AARON ZIMMERMAN

TABLE OF CONTENTS

INTRODUCTION

Vagus nerve stimulation is the use of a device to stimulate the vagus nerve with electrical impulses. The term vagus nerve stimulation further includes any technique that is used to stimulate the vagus nerve. You will wonder why you have to stimulate the vagus nerve at all. This is because vagus nerve stimulation may be the most suitable cure for recurrent seizures, cardiac failure, and other heart-related disorders that are unresponsive to medications. Vagus nerve stimulation has been proven to reduce the frequency of seizures, vasovagal syncope, depression, anxiety, stress, and several nervous system-related dysfunctions. Studies have shown that vagus nerve stimulation is helpful to people who haven't responded positively to intensive depression therapies, such as antidepressant medications, psychotherapy, and electroconvulsive therapy.

The Food and Drug Administration has approved vagus nerve stimulation for people over the age of four, and for those who have focal epilepsy and seizures that are non-responsive to medications. Vagus nerve stimulation has also been approved for alarming nervous disorders like vasovagal syncope, anxiety, stress, and depression. Adults with treatment-resistant depression can now take shield in vagus nerve stimulation. Standard therapies for these nervous system-related syndromes can be continued with vagus nerve stimulation. This way, the success of the treatment will be maximized.

Early observation of vagus nerve stimulation was first made in the 1880s when manual massage and compression of the carotid artery in the cervical region of the neck was effective in suppressing seizures. This effect was attributed to crude stimulation of the vagus nerve. Vagus nerve stimulation, if correctly done, is aimed at achieving soundness of the mind, improving vagal tone, correcting nervous related abnormalities, and, most of all, leaving you with a happier and healthier life. Isn't this something you should consider?

There are several ways of achieving vagus nerve stimulation. Most of the widely known methods involve the use of electrical impulses. In the conventional vagus nerve stimulation, a device is surgically implanted underneath the skin on your chest. A wire is threaded under your skin to the vagus nerve. The device is then activated, and electrical signals are sent through the cord to your vagus nerve. The most recent form is the use of noninvasive vagus nerve stimulation devices. This does not require surgical intervention to stimulate the vagus nerve. It has been approved by the Food and Drug Administration to take care of cluster headaches in the United States, and in the treatment of epilepsy, depression, and pain in Europe. Among these widely known methods are:

- The left cervical vagus nerve stimulation

- The right cervical vagus nerve stimulation

- Transcutaneous forms of vagus nerve stimulation

All these methods involve delivering electrical impulses straight to the vagus nerve, which have proven to be very useful. However, some studies have shown the side effects related to this method ranges from mild to severe. It is in the quest to avert this side effect that the crude way of stimulating the vagus nerve was improved on, to achieve the same effectiveness as the use of electrical impulses. This is what is now referred to as vagus nerve self-stimulation. In essence, vagus nerve self-stimulation is the natural method employed to spike the vagus nerve for effectiveness, without the use of any electrical devices.

Vagus nerve self-stimulation has successfully achieved the same effect as the clinical Vagus nerve stimulation. In other words, it can be used successfully with seizures, anxiety, stress, and depression therapies. Vagus nerve self-stimulation is conveniently used in the treatment of several nervous system abnormalities like vasovagal syncope, heart disorders, and improvement of the vagal tone. Vagus nerve self-stimulation is mostly preferred because it averts the risk of adverse events. It is safe, easy and can be practiced by every individual (including healthy people who are interested in improving their wellbeing), without any medical supervision. However, to effectively perform a vagus nerve self-stimulation, you need full knowledge of the nervous system and how it operates. This book has been penned down to guide you through that.

This beginner's guide simplifies the complexity of the nervous system and makes it an exciting and adventurous concept for everyone to understand. The vagus nerve should be your primary interest in the self-treatment of anxiety, stress, and depression. This is why this book guides you through the function and location of the vagus nerve. You need to understand the vagus nerve and know where it is before you can stimulate it. This beginner's guide also carries you through achieving success, with your self-therapy, that will hand you a happier and healthy life.

PART ONE

A HEALTHY LIFE LIES IN THE STATE OF YOUR BRAIN

CHAPTER ONE

UNDERSTANDING THE NERVOUS SYSTEM

To enjoy a healthy life, you must be conscious of the state of your nervous system. This tells you that the quality of life you get is directly proportional to the condition of your brain and spinal cord. The nervous system comprises of a complex network of nerves and specialized cells that communicate with the brain and every other part of the body. These nerves and cells transmit information to and from the brain and targeted organs or tissues. This information can also be referred to, in simple terms, as signals or stimuli. The nervous system is responsible to coordinate the actions of every part of the body in relation to its immediate environment. To increase the chances of survival, every living organism must react accordingly to environmental changes.

The regulation of these reactions is dependent solely on the nervous system, thus making the nervous system the most complicated of all body systems. Environmental change provides the external stimulus recognized by a receptor organ and transmitted to the central nervous system either through the peripheral nervous system or directly, depending on the site of stimulation.

Basic Functional Structures Of The Nervous System

The nervous system comprises of several vital structures for effective dissimilation of its functions. Some of these structures have been described in simple terms along with the functions of each. The understanding of these structures and their individual functions is important in identifying impairment. A slight deviation from the normal alignment of this structures can lead to abnormal performance or total loss of function of other organs and tissues innervated by the affected nerve.

The effector organs are responsible for the reaction or responses provoked in response to the external stimulation. The receptor organs translate every stimulus or signal to an electrical potential, regardless of the stimuli. The impulse travels in this coded form through a chain of neurons and ultimately ends in the efferent neuron to effect response. Neurons are therefore the basic unit from which the nervous system is created.

A neuron is an elongated cell constituting the cell body which contains the nucleus and various processes. These processes include the axon and dendrites. The diverse variety of neurons has specific distributions that are related to their specific functions. The unique structure of the neuron enables it to receive impulses from many different sources. Several synaptic connections are established to enable appropriate diffusion of the impulses.

A nerve impulse can be referred to as the action potential. The action potential arriving at the presynaptic junction of the axon does not jump from one cell to the next, rather, it moves through an organized mechanism by releasing specific chemical transmitter substances that diffuse through the synapse to produce its effect. The produced effect can either be to depolarize the membrane or to hyperpolarize the membrane. If a membrane is depolarized, a fresh impulse is initiated and is propagated through the length of the postsynaptic cell. If the membrane is hyperpolarized, an inhibitory effect is produced.

Sometimes, both excitatory and inhibitory effects can be established on the same cell, thus providing a means for a great diversity of responses. There are several transmitter substances, the most common being acetylcholine, glycine, noradrenaline, and serotonin. Neurons are not just an independent structure of their own. They are supported by several specialized cells. The supporting tissues of the brain and spinal cord are called the neuroglia. The neuroglia comprises of several cell types.

Aside from their supportive function, the neuroglia cells assist in the nutrition of the neurons and provide the nerve fibers of the brain and spinal cord with rich cytoplasmic investment that insulates these fibers from their surroundings. The neuroglia cells are therefore important to prevent leakages of the impulses these fibers convey. The insulating material of the nerve fibers in the central nervous system is known as myelin. It is common to represent these nerves as a whitish connection of fibers. This is because the myelin incidentally imparts a whitish color to the nerve fibers. The brain and spinal cord are also enclosed in a series of connective tissue segments that are referred to as the meninges.

Nerve fibers within the peripheral trunk receive a very similar form of insulation of varying thickness from a different type of supporting structure known as the Schwann cell. Schwann cells are also referred to as the neurolemmocytus. There are also connective tissue segments that further protect and support the peripheral nerve trunk. The peripheral nerve trunks are subdivided by these connective tissue sheaths and septa. The brain and spinal cord however are not penetrated or subdivided by connective tissues.

Fiber bundles are aggregated within the brain and spinal cord into a tracts or fasciculi. The spinocerebellar tracts and the cerebellospinal tracts are typical examples of this fasciculi. The neuronal aggregations upon the peripheral nerves may form visible swellings and are universally called the ganglia.

The Stimulus-Response Apparatus

The stimulus-response apparatus is concerned with the relationship between a stimulus and a reaction. The simplest form of response is the direct one-to-one stimulus-response reaction. Stimulus-response apparatus accounts for conditioning, coordination, behavior, and the general performance of a person. A change in the environment is a typical stimulus, and your reaction to this change is the response. Responses involve the synchronization and integration of a series of events in different parts of the human body. A controlled mechanism is located between the stimulus and the response initiated. The two basic mechanisms by which integration is achieved are referred to as the chemical regulation and the nervous regulation.

The chemical regulation employs the use of certain substances called hormones to initiate responses. Hormones are produced by a group of well-defined cells that are either diffused or carried via the bloodstream to the targeted tissues where they can now effect changes. Hormones perform several functions in the body: they can influence metabolism and induce the synthesis of other substances. Changes resulting from hormonal actions are expressed in the body as "influences on" or "alteration in" form, growth, reproduction, and behavior.

The nervous regulation of stimulus-response coordination integrates their effect through neurons. The neurons are a group of specialized cells designed deliberately for the conduction of impulses. Impulses are commonly described as the "excited state." An excitation produced by a stimulus travels from a sensory receptor to the brain. It returns with the "effect" through a more extensive network of nerves to an effector, which is the site at which the response is initiated. Considering the complexity of the nervous system, isn't it amazing how rapidly responses are initiated?

The body is very much organized in such a way that any stimuli that tends to disrupt part of the body's normal functioning calls for an immediate response that results in the reduction of the adverse effects of such stimuli and a return to more normal conditioning. The stimuli-response cascade also influences behavioral patterns and is vital to the adaptive ability of every individual. Although stimuli-response coordination is beneficial to an individual, it is not always performed consciously in response to a person's need or stimulus. Most of the stimulus-response coordination covers involuntary responses to stimuli. It is important to mention that learned behavior can be superimposed on both homeostatic regulation and some of the nervous system functions.

Aaron Zimmerman

Arrangement Of The Stimulus-Response Apparatus

The stimulus-response apparatus is made of four elements arranged in series: a receptor, an afferent neuron, a synapse, and an effector. The receptor region's function is to respond to stimuli of a specific modality. These stimuli can be sound, touch and pain related to environmental changes. These impulses can be perceived in the cells in various ways depending on their intensity, duration and frequency of delivery, and thus produce electrical, chemical and/or mechanical changes. The afferent neuron region conveys each impulse centrally towards the brain or the spinal cord. The synapse reminds the efferent neuron to convey impulse from the center to the periphery. The last in the series is the effector. The effector may be muscles, glands or neurosecretory cells where the effect of the stimulus will be expressed instantaneously.

The arrangement further constitutes the primary, elementary or monosynaptic reflex arc. The stretch reflex is a well-known type of monosynaptic reflex arc in which the muscles, muscle spindles and other receptors within the muscle and tendons are stretched. The impulse moves through the afferent nerve fibers to reach the central nervous system where it is projected towards the efferent nerves to initiate a typical muscle stretch. In most other reflexes, one or more additional neurons are interposed between the afferent and efferent neurons. These neurons are conveniently named interneurons. This kind of branching of the neurons enables a more refined control of activities upon consciousness.

The branching pathways are involved in securing that responses extend through several segments of the spinal cord. They reach and excite or inhibit the efferent neurons that supply various muscles through considerable stretches of the spinal cord. In order to maintain balance, coordination of these changes involves the higher centers within the brain. Messages must ascend to the higher centers in addition to the integration within the spinal cord. This process is most likely to be noticed by the individual. A person can assess a situation and determine whether a more general response like the flight or retaliation against the aggressor would be most appropriate. The flight or fight response is a far cry from the simple, monosynaptic, and monosegmental response of the stretch receptors. It involves integrative apparatuses of various degrees of complexity spreading through the spinal cord and brain, and draws upon those higher centers that are specifically concerned with memory and judgment.

THE DIVISIONS OF THE NERVOUS SYSTEM

In reality, the nervous system forms a single integrated whole. However, it is convenient and necessary to split it into parts. Understanding of the structural components of the nervous system, described in previous pages, will give you a good grab of the divisions of the nervous system. The most fundamental divisions being the central nervous system and the peripheral nervous system. The central nervous system consists of the brain and the spinal cord also called the neural axis. Every information comes to the central nervous system and also leaves from the central nervous system. An essential function of the central nervous system is the storage of this information. Information can be stored in the brain for many years. This is very much distinct from the peripheral nervous system, which is composed of the cranial, spinal, and the autonomic nerve trunks with their associated ganglia. It is termed the periphery to include every other part outside the brain and spinal cord. This division greatly facilitates description.

A further division in regards to function is based on the direction of the impulses and on the nature of information these impulses convey. This distinguishes the afferent systems from the efferent systems, both of which are subdivisions of the peripheral nervous system. The afferent system receives information from the surrounding environment and takes these impulses towards the spinal cord and then to the brain. The efferent system, on the other hand, takes these processed impulses from the brain either through the spinal cord or directly to the effector organ where this information is initiated. In essence, impulses move from the peripheral nervous system through the afferent pathway to the central nervous system for integration. Then it is taken back from the central nervous system through the peripheral nervous system (this time through the efferent pathway) for initiation. You would not be wrong to describe the peripheral nervous system as a pathway and the central nervous system as the processor of these signals.

Since the afferent pathway has the sensation functions, it is conveniently named the sensory divisions of the nervous system. Here, the information travels from the periphery towards the brain or spinal cord through the sensory nerves. Within the spinal cord, it is often described as the ascending pathway. This description accommodates the characteristic of the impulses to travel from the lower ascending parts to the higher ascending parts towards the brain. The sensory nerves perceive varying degrees of sensations. These sensations cover every stimulus there is to be received from the environment. The environment can be either external or internal. The external environment comprises of everything happening outside the body, a typical example being the heat felt from the sun, flame, and electricity. In contrast, the internal environment covers everything happening within the body, with a typical example being heat from muscular activity.

The group of sensations detected by the afferent pathways is collectively termed the special senses. This includes stimuli detected by all the sense organs like the eyes, nose, ears, tongue, and skin. These stimuli are sight, smell, taste, touch, nociception and temperature. They are all detected by their individual receptors. The sensory branch of the nervous system is carefully grouped into two separate parts: the somatic part and the visceral part. The somatic part carries the somatic sensory information. Somatic sensory information are those signals that arise from the sensory receptors in the skin, skeletal muscles, or joints. The visceral part bares the visceral sensory information, which is information that arises from the sensory receptors in the blood vessels or internal organs.

The efferent pathway, on the other hand, initiates responses to those impulses: this is described as the motor function and is conveniently named the motor division of the nervous system. Information is received from the brain and spinal cord through the motor neurons. Impulses are conducted from the higher parts and lower parts of the brain and spinal cord to the periphery. Little wonder, the system is termed the descending or motor division. However, many descending fiber bundles are not motor bundles; likewise, many ascending fiber bundles are not sensory. The motor nerves receive processed impulses from the brain and spinal cord and take them to the targeted tissues where responses are initiated. The motor nerves initiate two types of responses, the voluntary responses, and involuntary responses. This constitutes the somatic nervous system and the autonomic nervous system respectively.

The somatic nervous system deals with dissimilating voluntary responses. The voluntary responses are purposeful responses. The somatic motor coordinates voluntary responses. Interestingly, the somatic motor only innervates the skeletal muscles. This means that voluntary actions are performed strictly by the skeletal muscles. If you are going to eat, your hands, your mouth, and your eyes are innervated by the somatic motor to pick up your meal, take a bite and chew. You can also decide not to eat. These actions are performed purposely. The decision to eat or not to eat was solely made by you. To carry out your decision, you need the assistance of the nerves. The nerves stimulate your muscles to go ahead with your decision to eat. If the nerve responsible for stimulating the muscles in your hands is paralyzed, you will not be able to pick up your food despite having an intact muscle. In the same way, if the nerves stimulating your mouth are paralyzed, you cannot chew the food in your mouth. This is how vital nerves are to your everyday activities. Voluntary responses are responses that you solely decide to make but are dependent on the wellness of your nerves for the initiation of these responses. The somatic system is, therefore, concerned with those functions that determine the relationship of an individual with its environment — functions like locomotion, eating and more.

Other muscles do not depend on your decision for the activation of their functions. This is the group of muscles concerned with involuntary actions. Involuntary actions are the second group of responses the body is subjected to daily. Involuntary responses do not require your recognition to go ahead with their effects. The responses happen without your control, and as such they are automatic responses. It is, therefore, very convenient that the autonomic motor nerves control them. The autonomic motor nerves innervate the cardiac muscles and smooth muscle (glandular tissues). The autonomic nervous system is solely responsible for involuntary responses. The movement of food through your bowel is not determined by your decision to take food up and down your gut but on the actions of the smooth muscle tissues lining your bowel. In the same way, you cannot determine the metabolism of the drugs your swallow purposely. The autonomic nervous system is concerned with functions that relate to the internal environment. It regulates the vascular system, heart rate, glandular activities, digestive process and more. It controls the fight or flight responses and the rest and digest response of every individual. Nonetheless, the somatic and autonomic systems work in close relation to effectively coordinate their individual functions.

THE AUTONOMIC NERVOUS SYSTEM

To adequately perform a vagus nerve self-stimulation, you need a full understanding of the autonomic nervous system. This is why we will dwell more on this topic. The autonomic nervous system is a branch of the peripheral nervous system. It was formerly referred to as the vegetative nervous system or the visceral nervous system and is connected only to the motor branch of the peripheral nervous system. The autonomic nervous system is a specially controlled system that acts largely unconsciously. Several body functions such as heart rate, respiratory rate, digestion, pupillary responses, urination and even sexual arousal are controlled by the autonomic nervous system. Nerves of the autonomic nervous system supply the smooth muscle and glands. In essence, they influence the functions of the internal organs. The autonomic nervous system is the primary mechanism involved in the control of the fight or flight responses and also the rest and digest responses.

Within the brain, the hypothalamus regulates the activities of the autonomic nervous system. Autonomic activities like respiration are controlled by the respiration control center of the hypothalamus, cardiac regulation by the cardiac control center, and vasomotor activity by the vasomotor center. Reflex activity such as coughing, sneezing, swallowing and vomiting are also supervised by the hypothalamic centers responsible for each. The hypothalamus acts as an integrator for autonomic functions by receiving regulatory input of the autonomic nervous system from the limbic system. The autonomic nervous system branches off to include the sympathetic nervous system, the parasympathetic nervous system, and of course, the enteric nervous system.

The enteric nervous system is not so much of a concern to this study since its function is confined to the gastrointestinal tract. However, it is good that we spell out clearly the characteristic function of the enteric nervous system. The enteric nervous system governs the functions of the gastrointestinal tract. It is made up of a group of a mesh-like system of neurons that help oversee this function. The enteric nervous system is totally capable of acting independently of the sympathetic and parasympathetic nervous systems, although it may be influenced by their actions. It is regarded as a second brain because of its independent nature. The enteric nervous system developed from the neural crest cells and is embedded in the lining of the gastrointestinal tract. Little wonder it is capable of operating independently of the brain and spinal cord. However, the enteric nervous system relies on innervations from the autonomic nervous system through the vagus nerve and the prevertebral ganglia in a healthy individual for effective functioning. Nonetheless, the enteric system is capable of performing its functions solely when the vagus nerve is in good shape.

The sympathetic nervous system is most active during sporting activities. Activities like running, jogging, and other exercises. You will notice that during these activities you breathe faster, grasp for air and sweat a lot. These are all sympathetic regulations to help you adjust to your current activity. The sympathetic nervous system is also active in horrific situations. When watching a horror movie, for instance, your heart rate increases rapidly, your eyes dilate widely as you are unsure of what to expect next and you are terrified of the unknown. This is your sympathetic system totally at work, preparing your body for the shock.

All these expressions of fear and anxiety can be seen when you hear a loud, terrifying sound, maybe from a gunshot or when faced with an enemy. Your airways will automatically be dilated, your heart rate and respiratory rate increased, your eyes wide open, and you would start to sweat profusely. Then you would begin to consider which options are best for you: would you be better-off avenging the attack? Or running as fast as your adrenalin can take you? Whatever it is, your sole aim is to disappear from this unfavorable situation unhurt.

All these calculations and actions occur within the blink of an eye, and you almost wouldn't notice you had considered your actions. This is why the sympathetic responses are classified as the fight or the flight response. Thus, the sympathetic system can appropriately be regarded as the "fight or flight" system. The complex of responses expressed during a fight or flight response mechanism is aimed at preparing the body for the worst. Dilation of the eyes widens your vision, so you can see more clearly during the fight or flight episode. Your airways are dilated so that you take in more air needed for the flight. You might also have noticed that the muscles around your belly and chest area tighten during a terrifying situation. This is not because these muscles love to constrict when you are nervous or because fear lives here, but because your sympathetic nervous system is located within this region. This means that most of the neurons that get you ready for the fight or flight episode come from your thoracic region and some of them also come from the lumber area. This describes your trunk or abdominal and thorax area. It is, therefore, convenient to say your sympathetic nerves arise from the thoracolumbar region.

The parasympathetic nervous system, on the other hand, is active during rest. The parasympathetic nervous system is considered as the "rest and digest" system. This system has an opposite action to the sympathetic system. Where one of the systems activates a physiological response, the other inhibits the specific action. The sympathetic system is a quick response mobilizing system; the parasympathetic system is a more slowly activated system. The parasympathetic system coordinates metabolism and other metabolic processes. While you are sleeping or simply relaxing, the parasympathetic system predominates over the activity of your body system. The parasympathetic system arises from the craniosacral outflow, which is above and below the sympathetic system. This describes the location of the parasympathetic nervous system, showing that some part of the system arises from the cranial nerves and the remaining part from the sacral nerves. Inhibitory and excitatory synapses occur between neurons. This makes the autonomic nervous system unique. The autonomic nervous system requires a sequential two-neuron efferent pathway. These are the preganglionic neuron and the postganglionic neuron. The preganglionic neuron begins the autonomic outflow and will first synapse the postganglionic neuron, which will then synapse at the effector organ for initiation of each response. All these responses occur very fast and without notice.

How The Autonomic Nervous System Works

The autonomic nervous system is one of the most vital parts of the nervous system. It regulates a variety of body processes without conscious effort. The autonomic nervous system is responsible for body functions such as heartbeat, blood flow, breathing, and digestion. Aside from the fight or flight responses of the sympathetic nervous system, it is responsible for tasks like relaxing the bladder, dilating the eye pupils and speeding up the heart rate. In general, the sympathetic system prepares for activity, providing more glucose so you can have sufficient energy, and prevents the activity of digestion because you wouldn't need your blood glucose to be stored at such times. The parasympathetic nervous system is known for its relaxing function. It helps conserve physiological resources like preventing unnecessary loss of energy. It conserves your hard earn energy for more useful times. It is also responsible for maintaining normal body functions. It facilitates digestion, stimulates digestive secretions, and increases gut mobility. It goes further to control the bladder, constrict the eye pupils, and of course, slow down the heart rate.

We have now seen that the autonomic nervous system works by the opposing effect of the sympathetic and parasympathetic systems. When the sympathetic system stimulates a response, the parasympathetic inhibits it and vice versa. The sympathetic system is believed to be the quick responding system that mobilizes the body system for immediate action, but the parasympathetic system acts much more slowly to dampen responses. So, if the sympathetic nervous system raises blood pressure, the parasympathetic nervous system will go ahead to lower blood pressure. By working together this way, the autonomic nervous system can manage body functions appropriately. Imagine if the blood pressure was left elevated permanently with no relaxing responses to lower it. The blood pressure would remain elevated and possibly continue to rais until the body can no longer bear. To prevent this, it is appropriate that we have a soothing and opposing effect on each body response.

The sympathetic and parasympathetic systems work together to manage body responses depending on the immediate situation or body needs. This is termed the dual autonomic innervation. Although there are exceptions to this, most organs are innervated by the branches of the autonomic system. Like it was stated earlier, if you are facing a treat and need to flee from or avenge the treat, the sympathetic system immediately mobilizes your body for this. Once the treatment is over, as you obviously cannot remain in that mood forever, the parasympathetic system steps in and takes over the sympathetic from here, dampening those responses, and slowly returning your body to its normal resting state. The autonomic nervous system coordinates the following internal processes;

- Digestions

- Blood pressure

- Pupillary responses

- Heart rate

- Respiratory rate

- Emotional responses

- Sexual responses

- Metabolism

- Body temperature

- Electrolyte balance

- Urination and defecation

- Production of body fluids, including sweat and saliva.

You would wonder what else it is that the autonomic nervous system doesn't control. It controls varieties of critical internal body processes. This makes the autonomic system very special. This does not intend to scare you, but the truth is any alteration to this system and its parts can be very severe and life-threatening. This is why you should learn how to safeguard your nervous system and, of course, manage stress, anxiety, and depression appropriately to live a healthy life.

How Impulses Travel From Central Nervous System Through The Autonomic Nervous System Then To The Target Tissues

The autonomic nervous system coordinates its functions through the autonomic nerve pathways. The autonomic nerve pathways connect different organs to the brain stem and spinal cord. The brain stem is the posterior part of the brain, and it houses ten cranial nerves. There are twelve cranial nerve cells in all and they will be further discussed in the following pages. Information is sent down the autonomic nerve pathways to the effector organ with the assistance of the neurotransmitters. Neurotransmitters are chemical messengers through which the autonomic nerves communicate. The two neurotransmitters that are important for communication within the autonomic nervous system are acetylcholine and norepinephrine.

As said in the earlier pages of this book, nerve cells synapse with one another at the ganglions. In the sympathetic system, nerve cells are coming out of the spinal cord and then synapse at the ganglion, and new nerve cells will then target the effector tissues. There are several sympathetic ganglions. In the parasympathetic system, the nerve cells arise from the brain stem and the sacral region of the spinal cord would synapsing different ganglions before being transmitted to a new nerve cell, which will then target the effector organ. These nerve cells are conveniently called the pre- and postganglionic neurons. The arrangement is such that the preganglionic neuron comes out of the brain or spinal cord and synapses at the ganglion and the postganglionic synapse at the other end of the ganglion picks the information and transmits it to the receptor cells of the effector organ. The preganglionic neuron of the sympathetic nervous system is short and lightly myelinated while its postganglionic neuron is long and unmyelinated. In the parasympathetic system, the preganglionic neuron is long and myelinated while the postganglionic neuron is short and unmyelinated. This design is purposeful and can give a little explanation as to why responses from the sympathetic system are more rapid than those of the parasympathetic.

Action potential travels from the axon of the preganglionic neuron to reach the axon terminal where neurotransmitters are released. All the preganglionic neurons of the autonomic system are cholinergic. This means that they all produce and release acetylcholine. Therefore, the neurotransmitter produced by the preganglionic neurons is the acetylcholine. In the parasympathetic and somatic nervous system, the postganglionic neurons are also cholinergic, which means that after synapse at the presynaptic junction and release of acetylcholine by the preganglionic neuron, the postganglionic neurons continue with the production and release of acetylcholine at the nerve terminals. Whereas, at the sympathetic system, the postganglionic neuron is adrenergic. It, therefore, produces and releases norepinephrine. Cholinergic receptors are found in several places, both on the dendrites or cell body and effector organs innervated by the parasympathetic system. They are called the nicotinic 2 receptors and muscarinic receptors, respectively. The adrenergic receptors located on the effector organs innervated by the sympathetic nervous system can either be the alpha receptors or the beta receptors. Epinephrine (adrenaline) is released from the adrenal glands to bind with the adrenergic receptors on the effector organ and activate it. The receptor organ would thus become sensitive to the norepinephrine released.

Finally, information is transmitted through the parasympathetic nerves through the cranial nerves and sacral branch of the spinal nerves. In the sympathetic nervous system, impulses are transmitted through the spinal nerves. There are thirty-one spinal nerves and twelve cranial nerves. We will focus on the cranial nerves. The twelve cranial nerves include:

- Cranial nerve one is the olfactory nerve, which is a sensory nerve. It travels through the ethmoid bone and lay upon the cribriform plate. It receives sensory information from the environment and takes them to the brain.

- Cranial nerve two is the optic nerve, which is also a sensory nerve. They receive information on vision from the retina and send them to the brain.

- Cranial nerve three is the oculomotor nerve is a motor nerve. It arises from the midbrain. It supplies most of the muscle of the eyeballs (the rectus and oblique muscles). It also innervates the ciliary muscles of the eye, and so, your oculomotor nerve is vital for accommodation.

- Cranial nerve four is the trochlear nerve. It is also a motor nerve, and it arises from the midbrain. It also supplies one of the eyeball muscles (the superior oblique).

- Cranial nerve five is the trigeminal nerve. It performs both the sensory and motor function; it can, therefore, be innervated by both the sensory division of the peripheral nervous system and the motor division. It is a very big nerve that is responsible for most of the facial sensation. It originates from the pons and the midbrain and has three branches (ophthalmic, maxillary, and the mandibular).

- Cranial nerve six is the abducent nerve. It also arises from the pons and is also responsible for the eyeball movement. It is a motor nerve for the lateral rectus muscles of the eye.

- Cranial nerve seven is the facial nerve. It performs both sensory and motor function and originates from the pons. As the name suggests, it supplies the face. It is responsible for the muscles of facial expression. It also supplies all the secretory glands of your face (the lacrimal glands for tears production and much more). It also innervates the anterior two-thirds of the tongue for taste.

- Cranial nerve eight is the vestibulocochlear nerve. It is a sensory nerve that branches off into two parts. The vestibular nerve comes from the vestibule of the inner ear and the cochlear nerves which come off the cochlear. They join and form the vestibulocochlear nerve, which travels to the pons area of the brain.

- Cranial nerve nine is the glossopharyngeal nerve; it has both the sensory and motor function and takes its origin from the medulla. It performs the tasting function.

- Cranial nerve ten is the vagus nerve. It originates from the medulla oblongata and performs both the sensory and motor function. Vagus nerve is the nerve of the fourth and subsequent pharyngeal arches. It constitutes the parasympathetic fibers that innervate the cervical, the thoracic, and abdominal viscera. Little wonder, it controls several organs in the body, specifically the digestive organs. The vagus nerve is responsible for stimulating the rest and digests response, which is the opposite of the fight or flight response that you have heard so much about.

- Cranial nerve eleven is the accessory nerve. It performs the motor function and also originates from the medulla.

- Cranial nerves twelve is the hypoglossal nerve. It originates from the medulla and performs the motor function, basically for the movement of the tongue.

Each of these cranial nerves perform much more than the functions stated above. This is basically to give you a general overview of the functions of the parasympathetic nervous system and most importantly, the *vagus nerve*. We have seen that the vagus nerve innervates most of the organs in the body, including the heart, the lungs, the stomach, intestines, liver, kidneys, urethras and all the other organs within the trunk. The sympathetic nervous system also innervates the same organs within the trunk through the spinal nerves, but in a different way from the parasympathetic system. This lays the basis for the opposing effect of the sympathetic and parasympathetic nervous system.

GETTING TO KNOW YOUR VAGUS NERVE

The word vagus was coined from a Latin word, meaning wandering. This should give you a quick idea of how vastly the vagus nerve can travel. The vagus nerve is your major concern when embarking on a nerve stimulation therapy. The vagus nerve extends from the brainstem down through your cervical region to your thorax. It further extends into your abdominal region on both sides of your body. As it travels, the vagus nerve innervates organs in all these regions. This tells you how long this nerve must be. It wanders through your viscera, innervating each of them as it goes. It supplies the muscles of your face and neck and goes further to innervate your heart, lungs, and down to your gut, supplying your stomach and intestines. As stated earlier, the vagus nerve is one of the cranial nerves of the parasympathetic nervous system. The vagus nerve is, of course, the reason why the rest and digest function is recognized as the major function of the parasympathetic system. The vagus nerve is critical for the treatment of mental health conditions. The vagus nerve is also a key player in your gut instinct: it does this through the body-mind connection it creates. The knot in your throat and the sparkles in your smile is all due to the effect of the vagus nerve. The vagus nerve is a two-way communication tool: it helps you stay in touch with your senses and emotions by giving meaning to your thoughts through your displayed behavior. Deep down your gut, you know it now! The vagus nerve is the big guy that controls your mood from the inside! But how does it achieve this? Why not stick around to find out.

CHAPTER TWO

WHEN THE BODY MALFUNCTIONS

The primary cause of several diseases we see in society today can be traced down to the disorganization and dysfunction of the body cells. The body is a complex organization of cells designed in a way to cater for itself. However, some of these cells can malfunction due to certain environmental triggers. Most of the factors that may provoke the disorganization of these cells result from the misbehavior of the cells themselves. The cells may either perform their functions below normal or even over the usual. Either way, an alarm will be raised by other regulatory cells to subject the body to check. This signal travels to and from the nervous system. This is how the body maintains orderliness and keeps you safe and healthy. Problems arise when the body can no longer effectively manage itself. What happens next, when the body cells malfunction?

Aaron Zimmerman

CHOLINERGIC ANTI-INFLAMMATORY PATHWAY

Malfunctioning of the body cells disturbs homeostasis. This disturbance to homeostasis can result from an injury, infection or trauma, which will result in inflammation. Inflammation is the normal way our bodies respond to disturbed homeostasis through a complex series of immune reactions to neutralize the invading pathogens, repair injured tissues and promote wound healing. The release of pro-inflammatory mediators characterizes the onset of inflammations. These mediators are cells that destroy the disturbing pathogen and bring the body back to its normal state. The mediators include macrophages, interleukin (IL)-1, tumor necrosis factor (TNF), adhesion molecules, vasoactive mediators and reactive oxygen species. The early release of pro-inflammatory cytokines by activated macrophages has a vital role in triggering local inflammatory response. However, excessive production of these cytokines can be more injurious than the inciting event. If the cytokines are in excess, it can initiate diffuse coagulation, hypotension, tissue injury, and death.

To prevent this, inflammatory responses are balanced by anti-inflammatory factors like cytokines IL-10 and IL-4, IL-1 receptor antagonists and the transforming growth factor. Aside from the involvement of the TNF and IL-1β in local inflammation, they are signals for activation of brain-derived neuroendocrine immunomodulatory responses. The neuroendocrine pathways, like the sympathetic division of the autonomic nervous system and the hypothalamo-pituitary-adrenal (HPA) axis, controls inflammation as an anti-inflammatory balancing mechanism. In essence, the host mobilizes the immunomodulatory resources of the nervous and endocrine systems to regulate inflammation.

The usual restoration of homeostasis as a normal resolution of inflammation might not always occur. Insufficient inflammatory responses might lead to an increase in the body's susceptibility to infections and cancer. Excessive responses, on the other hand, can predispose the body to autoimmune diseases like sepsis, diabetes and other debilitating conditions. The loss of control of inflammatory responses is sequelae to the spilling of pro-inflammatory mediators into circulation. This may result in systemic inflammation that may progress to shock, multiple organ failure and, of course, death. To avert these complications, effective therapies to cater for diseases of excessive inflammation are required.

Studies have recently shown the anti-inflammatory action of the vagus nerve in an animal model with endotoxemia and shock. This previously unrecognized immunomodulatory circuit was conveniently termed cholinergic anti-inflammatory pathway. The brain can modulate systemic and local inflammation through cholinergic anti-inflammatory pathway. The Cholinergic anti-inflammatory pathway is a mechanism for neural inhibition of inflammation. It interfaces the brain with the immune system. This is only a concern with the brain-derived control mechanism of the immune function and the role of cholinergic anti-inflammatory pathway in the regulation of inflammation. The immune system and the brain interact closely to respond to immune-related challenges effectively. This is what the cholinergic anti-inflammatory pathway seeks to express.

Effective communication between the nervous, immune, and endocrine systems is essential for appropriate host defense against invading pathogens. The host defense usually involves a variety of mediators, including neurotransmitters, cytokines, hormones and humoral factors. The influence of the brain on immune functions and the mechanisms involved in these interactions have long been questioned. Question raising through the minds of scientist when describing the brain-derived immunomodulation are usually centered around how the brain is initially signaled by cytokines to trigger corresponding neural and neuroendocrine responses and on how the immunomodulation is achieved through these mechanisms. It is, therefore, essential to consider the immune-to-brain communications and the brain-to-immune communications and their impact on body cells.

Immune To Brain Communication

This is the medium through which the brain monitors the immune status and detects peripheral inflammation. It can achieve this adequately through two major pathways designated as the neural pathway and the humoral pathway. These pathways provide evidence of the vagus nerve as an immune check and modulator of good health and wellness.

The Neural Pathway

The neural pathway sends information to the brain that inflammation is occurring somewhere in the body. It relies on the activation of the vagus nerve afferent sensory fibers to signal the brain. Immunogenic impulses activate the vagus afferent fibers either directly through cytokines released from dendritic cells, macrophages and other vagal related immune cells, or indirectly through chemoreceptive cells located in vagal paraganglia. Intraperitoneal administration of endotoxin can induce IL-1β immunoreactivity in dendritic cells and macrophages within the connective tissues associated with the abdominal vagus nerve and in the subsequent vagal paraganglia and afferent fibers.

The visceral vagus afferent fibers, which reside in the nodose ganglion, terminate just within the dorsal vagal complex of the medulla oblongata. The dorsal vagal complex consists of the nucleus tractus solitarius, the area postrema and the dorsal motor nucleus of the vagus bundle. The dorsal motor nucleus is the major site of origin of the preganglionic vagus efferent fibers. The cardiovascular vagal efferent fibers also originate within the medullar nucleus ambiguous. The area postrema is a vital circumventricular organ and site for humoral immune-to-brain communication and it lacks a blood-brain barrier. The most important part of the vagal sensory input is received by neurons in the nucleus tractus solitarius that coordinates autonomic function and interaction with the endocrine system. Impulses ascending from the nucleus tractus solitarius reach the forebrain, hypothalamic nuclei, amygdala, and insular cortex. The paraventricular nuclei, which syntheses and releases corticotropin-releasing hormone (CRH) is one of the hypothalamic nuclei that receives this input coming from the nucleus tractus solitarius. The corticotropin releasing hormone is a very important substance in the hypoyhalamo-pituitary adrenal axis. This ascending link between the nucleus tractus solitarius and the paraventricular nuclei provides a pathway that can conveniently modulate neurohormonal anti-inflammatory responses.

A vast variety of synaptic contacts exist between the neurons in the nucleus tractus solitarius and C1 neurons in the rostral ventrolateral medulla. The rostral ventrolateral medulla occupies an important role in the control of cardiovascular homeostasis. The rostral ventricular medulla projects this signals to the locus coeruleus, which is the major source of noradrenergic innervations of higher brain sites, including the hypothalamus and paraventricular nuclei. Projections emanate from the rostral ventrolateral medulla and locus coeruleus to sympathetic preganglionic neurons in the spinal cord. Descending pathways from the paraventricular nuclei to the rostral ventrolateral medulla and nucleus tractus solitarius also exist. Each ascending and descending connections provides a neuronal substrate for the interaction between the hypothalamo-pituitary adrenal axis and the sympathetic nervous system as an immunomodulatory mechanism. Regardless of the integrity of the vagus nerve, transmission of cytokine signals to the brain through the vagal sensory neurons greatly depends on the magnitude of the immune challenge. The vagal afferent neural pathway is believed to play a dominant role in the mild to moderate peripheral inflammatory responses. A robust or acute inflammatory response signals the brain primarily through the humoral pathway.

The Humoral Pathway

Cases of systemic immune challenge largely provide evidences of the involvement of the humoral mechanisms in the immune to brain communication. The circulating cytokines released during inflammation are able to communicate with the brain structures involved in the anti-inflammatory response. The circulating cytokines are able to induce central cytokine production associated with fever and illness. Apart from their role in signaling the brain for immunomodulatory responses, cytokines play a multifunctional role in brain injury and neurodegenerative diseases. The blood borne IL-1β and tumor necrosis factor (TFN) are able to cross the blood brain barrier and enter the cerebrospinal fluid and interstitial fluid spaces of the brain and spinal cord by a saturable carrier-mediated mechanism, which may function only at a very high plasma cytokine concentration. Cytokines can also bind to surface receptors at the endothelium of the brain capillaries to enhance the synthesis and release of soluble mediators like prostaglandins and nitric oxide. This soluble mediator diffuses into the brain parenchyma to regulate the activity of specific groups of neurons. Prostaglandins are also believed to regulate fever and hypothalamo-pituitary axis activation.

Another way that cytokine-to-brain communication occurs is through the circumventricular organs which lack normal blood-brain barrier function. The area postrema, among all other circumventricular organs appears to lead the transduction site for the cytokine to brain communication through circumventricular organs. The area postrema is located on the floor of the caudal 4th ventricle and dendrites of neurons in the nucleus tractus solitarius and dorsal motor nucleus of the vagus bundle. The arrangement of the pathway favors communication along with the sympathetic nervous system and hypothalamo-pituitary axis. Within the area postrema, nucleus tractus solitarius, and rostral ventrolateral medulla, cytokine induces production of prostaglandins, which may activate the catecholamine projections to the paraventricular nucleus, resulting in subsequent activation of the hypothalamo-pituitary axis. This summarizes the possible interactions between the neural and humoral mechanisms of immune to brain communication through which the brain effectively regulates anti-inflammatory responses.

Brain To Immune Communication

The brain exerts strong regulatory effects on the immune function by the activation of the hypothalamo-pituitary adrenal axis and the sympathetic nervous system. This results in increased production and release of glucocorticoids and catacholamines. The hypothalamo-pituitary adrenal axis is a neurohomonal pathway with a wide role in the regulation of immune function. The hypothalamic paraventricular nucleus, the anterior pituitary and the adrenal cortex make up the part of the hypothalamo-pituitary adrenal axis. There are specialized neurons in the paraventricular nucleus that synthesize corticotropin, releasing hormone and releasing it into the pituitary portal blood system. These specialized neurons also stimulate the synthesis of adrenocorticotropin hormone (ACTH) from the anterior pituitary. Adrenocorticotropin hormone then inhibits the synthesis of corticotropin-releasing hormone from the paraventricular nucleus. Adrenocorticotropin hormone is the main inducer of the synthesis and release of immunosuppressive glucocorticoids (cortisol) from the adrenal cortex. Pro-inflammatory cytokines trigger the hypothalamo-pituitary adrenal axis through the neural or humoral mechanisms, as described above. At both the hypothalamic and pituitary levels, the hypothalamo-pituitary adrenal axis is subject to a classical negative feedback loop by the final product, glucocorticoids. The hypothalamo-pituitary circuit of the hypothalamo-pituitary adrenal axis is regulated by neural mechanisms, including acetylcholine (ACh), catecholamine, GABA, serotonin, and histamine-mediated modulation.

Autonomic responses represent the interplay of both the sympathetic nervous system and the parasympathetic nervous system. The sympathetic nervous system plays a dual role in the regulation of inflammation by regulating both pro-inflammatory and anti-inflammatory activities. It is, therefore, an integral component of the host defense system against injury and infection. Within the adrenal glands, the sympathetic neural regulation is converted into hormonal regulation. Therefore, the adrenals are a critical peripheral component of the brain-controlled immunoregulation responsible for the synthesis of glucocorticoids (from the cortical cells) and catecholamines (from the medullar chromaffin cells). Activation of the sympathetic nervous system protects the cells against the detrimental effects of pro-inflammatory cytokines. The parasympathetic vagal efferent system also plays a vital role in immunomodulation. The cholinergic anti-inflammatory pathway entails the neural immunomodulatory mechanism of systemic and local inflammation through the influence of the vagus nerve. Lowering the biological threshold for stress can reduce inflammation. Therefore, reducing the fight or flight responses of the sympathetic system would facilitate healing. A reduction in sympathetic activity is achieved through an increase in parasympathetic activity, which can be achieved by stimulating the vagus nerve.

HEART RATE VARIABILITY

Do you ever wonder what the impact of a stressful day would be on your health? If you have stuck around with this book this far, you are interested in improving your ability to have a better day each morning. Monitoring your sleep, performance, and overall health should be your major concern. Understanding heart rate variability becomes your key to achieving total control of a healthy life. Studies have shown that higher heart rate variability is associated with reduced morbidity and mortality. Higher heart rate variability has also been shown to improve psychological well-being and quality of life.

What Then Is Heart Rate Variability?

Heart rate variability is the physiological theory of variation in the time interval between every heartbeat. The autonomic nervous system controls this variation. The hypothalamus is constantly processing information and sending this processed information to the other parts of the body through the autonomic nervous system to either stimulate or relax different functions. The hypothalamus is responsible not only for a poor night sleep or for sour interactions between your spouse, boss or friends, but also for the reactions to those exciting news you got engaged with or for the delicious meal you had for lunch. The brain handles all forms of stimulus life throws at it. However, if you have persistent stimulators like anxiety, stress, poor sleep, depression, unhealthy diet, isolation, fear, dysfunctional relationships or lack of exercise, the body balance may be disrupted, and your fight or flight response or relax and digest balance could shift into overdrive.

Heart rate variability can also be called cycle length variability or heart period variability. Heart rate variability is influenced by exercise, metabolic processes, hormonal reactions, stress, recovery and cognitive process. Reduced heart rate variability is a cause of death after myocardial infarction. Heart rate variability is closely related to emotional arousal. Individuals who worry too much have been shown to have low heart rate variability. Elevated heart rate variability is responsible for the happiness people feel; it guarantees a relaxed state of the body and effective regulation of the homeostasis.

Every form of healing has a place to perfect wellbeing. Heart rate variability is a form of healing that helps the body recover from constantly not being at ease to experiencing a total relaxed, healthy state. Heart rate variability monitors the inconsistent gaps between each heartbeat. This makes it suitable as an index of the influence of both the parasympathetic nervous system and the sympathetic nervous system. Every aspect of physiology represents the balance of these two influences. High heart rate variability represents proper emotional regulation, decision making, and the perfect attention we desire. Low heart rate variability reflects the opposite of all these.

The Autonomic Nervous System In Relation To The Heart Rate Variability

Actions of the autonomic nervous system are closely related to the degree of heart rate variability. The parasympathetic innervation of the heart works quickly to decrease heart rate while the sympathetic innervation slowly increases heart rate. This function comes to play in accordance with the physiological states of the body at every minute. An individual with high heart rate variability would, therefore, reflect increased parasympathetic activities and so would experience a more relaxed state of mind. The same goes for an individual with low heart rate variability, which will reflect more sympathetic activity and, therefore, experience a heart-racing activity that is characterized by nervousness all through the day.

Neurovisceral integration is a model of heart rate variability that describes the central autonomic network as the decision-maker of cognitive, behavioral, and physiological regulation as they relate to a continuum of emotion. The neurovisceral integration describes how the prefrontal cortex regulates the activities of the limbic structures acting to depress parasympathetic activity and activate sympathetic circuits. Variation in the output of these two divisions of the autonomic system produces heart rate variability. Activity in the prefrontal cortex can, therefore, modulate the heart rate of variability. Positive heart rate variability regulates our emotions, attention, and decision making. Each of these characteristics is positively activated by elevated heart rate variability. Heart rate variability accompanied by a poor physiological state like anxiety has been found to result in poor decisions. Improving your heart rate variability through vagus nerve stimulation will result in improved wellbeing and health.

CIRCADIAN RHYTHM

If you feel energized and drowsy at about the same time each day, you should thank your circadian rhythm. The circadian rhythm is a 24-hour internal clock. It runs in the background of your brain and cycles between sleepiness and alertness at a regular interval. Circadian rhythm describes the physical, mental, and behavioral changes that follow a daily cycle. It basically responds to light and darkness in the environment. Being awake during the day and sleeping at night typically speaks of the light-related circadian rhythm. Your circadian rhythm is your sleep or wake cycle. A part of the hypothalamus regulates the circadian rhythm. It can also be influenced by other factors like lightness and darkness. When it is dark, your eyes send a signal to the hypothalamus, saying it's time for you to feel tired. Your brain will, in turn, signal your body to release melatonin, which will make your body and mind tired. This is why it is difficult for you to stay awake at night.

A regular sleeping habit would promote the maximal index of your circadian rhythm. Going to bed at night and waking up in the morning at about the same time daily will promote your circadian rhythm. However, some factors can get in the way of your circadian rhythm. Growing older can affect your circadian rhythm. You may not have the same circadian rhythm as your spouse, child, or parent. Jet lag, your occupation, activities or illness can also get in the way of your circadian rhythm. When the circadian rhythm is disturbed, it might be challenging to pay attention during your daily activity. The strong frequency of your circadian rhythm is felt during wake times. When you are sleep-deprived is the only time you will notice stronger swings of sleepiness and alertness. If more attention is directed to your body, you will notice feelings of alertness and drowsiness. Developing good sleeping hygiene will maintain your circadian rhythm and make your life better.

EMOTION REGULATION

Emotion and attention regulation should also come into mind when discussing health and vitality. Maybe you always wondered why one moment you are happy and the next you are sad. We refer to this behavior as mood swings. However, this is your emotional self-regulation at work. Emotional regulation is the ability of every individual to respond to the ongoing demands of experience with a range of emotions in a way that is socially tolerable to permit spontaneous reactions. It is a complex process that involves initiating, inhibiting or controlling one's state or behavior in a given situation. Emotional regulation is a highly substantial part of human life. Emotional regulation is concerned with the accurate modulation of your feelings, thoughts, emotion-related physiological responses and behavior. It describes the tendency to focus your attention on a task and your ability to suppress inappropriate behavior. We are continually exposed to a wide variety of potentially arousing stimuli daily. Unchecked emotional reactions to such stimuli could impede a functional fit with society. Therefore, we must all engage in some form of emotional regulation at all times.

The inability to control the influences of emotional arousal on the organization and quality of thoughts, actions and interactions is conveniently termed emotional dysregulation. People who are emotionally dysregulated exhibit patterns of responding to the ongoing situation in such a manner that there is a mismatch between their goals, responses and modes of expression, with the demands of the social environment. Emotional dysregulation is closely associated with depression, anxiety, eating disorder, and substance abuse. High levels of emotion regulation are largely related to both high levels of social competence and appropriate expression of social emotions.

Emotions come from the time and impact of a situation on a person. The ability to effectively modulate your emotions is vital for your social wellbeing and environment. Heart rate variability provides a window to the physiological components associated with emotional regulation. Heart rate variability reflects emotional regulation at two different levels, while resting and when caught up in a task. An individual with higher heart rate variability while resting would provide more appropriate emotional responses when compared with those with lower heart rate variability. This is particular with negative emotions. Your heart rate variability is subjected to change in relation to your emotions. Attention regulation is equally as substantial as emotional regulation. Heart rate variability can also have an effect on attention. People with high anxiety and low heart rate variability tend to have poor concentration. Studies have shown that increased focus and emotional regulation are linked with elevated heart rate variability and vagus nerve activity.

VASOVAGAL SYNCOPE

It is no longer rare to see people slump in parks, shopping malls, and even in swimming pools. Have you ever wondered why? Fainting has increasingly become an issue of concern in today's society, with vasovagal syncope taking the lead in each fainting episode. It is necessary to mention that vasovagal syncope is sometimes referred to as the neurocardiogenic syncope. Vasovagal syncope is a syndrome that is characterized by fainting. It arises due to the body's overreaction to specific triggers. Triggers such as the sight of blood or extreme emotional distress are prominent factors that can predispose a person to vasovagal syncope. These triggers cause the heart rate and blood pressure to drop suddenly, which would, in turn, lead to reduced blood flow to the brain. This is sequelae to a brief loss of consciousness, resulting in actual fainting.

Vasovagal syncope is not usually harmful and does not necessarily require treatment. However, it is possible to injure oneself during a sudden vasovagal syncope episode. Therefore, it is important to take measures that will rule out more severe causes of fainting. Numerous factors can predispose one to vasovagal syncope. These factors range from several heart disorders to an extreme phobia for blood.

There are several symptoms of vasovagal syncope, among which are pale skin, impaired vision, nausea, sweating and abnormal movements. Recovery from a vasovagal syncope episode generally begins in less than a minute, notwithstanding the fact that getting up too soon leaves you at risk of another fainting episode. Fainting being the major sign of vasovagal syncope may also indicate other severe conditions such as a heart or brain disorder. This is why you must understand the concept of vasovagal syncope and seek the needed medical attention.

Understanding vasovagal syncope requires a fundamental knowledge of the nervous system. Any impairment in the activity of the vagus nerve can trigger vasovagal syncope. The part of the nervous system initiating normal heart rate and blood pressure can malfunction or overreact to triggers such as an unexpected sight of blood. Also, underlying disease conditions such as heart disorders and delays in therapy can result in complications. Other common triggers include standing for more extended periods than the body can bear, exposure to excessive heat, anxiety and straining. These triggers cause a sudden drop in the heart rate that is characteristic of the vasovagal syncope. The blood vessels of your legs dilate, allowing blood to pool in your legs. This instantly lowers blood pressure, slows the heart rate even further and reduces blood flow through your brain. Your body responds to this cascade of events by fainting. Vasovagal syncope is a condition associated with the autonomic nervous system that can be managed if prompt vagus nerve therapy is conducted.

If you feel you are going to faint the next minute, you can lie down immediately and lift your legs. This would allow a continuous flow of blood through your brain. If lying down is not convenient for you, you can avert fainting by sitting down and keeping your heads between your knees until you feel much better. Tricks like these will help restore the function of your parasympathetic nervous system. The cascade of events that rapidly takes place within the body before, during and after a vasovagal syndrome is in close relation to anxiety, stress and depression. This is why we will discuss in detail the effect of these conditions on your health in the following pages. We will also consider simple tricks that will help you avert anxiety, stress, and depression. Read on and get more tips on how to live your best.

CHAPTER THREE

ANXIETY, STRESS, AND DEPRESSION

The three mental health conditions of anxiety, stress and depression can greatly impact on our vagal tone. Therefore, if we want to stimulate our vagus nerve, we must pay attention to these states and how to minimize their effects on our bodies. In this chapter, we will discuss the effect of anxiety, stress and depression on vagus nerve stimulation and how to create calm when we are caught up in these states. Before venturing into this however, it is important that we get background knowledge of anxiety, stress and depression and how these conditions affect our lives.

Understanding Anxiety, Stress and Depression

Only about ten percent of people who suffer depression do so without any stress triggers. Many other people suffer depression that's related to stress. Depression has a wide range of causes as does anxiety and stress.

Sometimes, the causes can be positive things like getting married and starting a new job or a new career path. When a person experiences stress from positive situations, they can give way to both anxiety and depression. In many ways, stress can be a good thing. Stress comes with a pressure that drives us into productivity. Sometimes, it even improves our performance. When we face the stress that deadlines bring, we are forced to achieve our best within a short time. In this way, stress is good for us. As with everything else, it is too much stress that isn't good.

Stress can keep us alert and motivated but these two states are sadly not what we get when we are stressed out. When the stress that we encounter is too much, we become susceptible to several unhealthy conditions. One of those conditions is depression. Stress in its acute or chronic states can lead to major depression. We must guard against this. Esther Stenberg, MD, stress researcher and chief of neuroendocrine immunology and behavior at the National Institute of Mental Health, puts it this way, "Like email and email spam, a little stress is good but too much is bad; you'll need to shut down and reboot." Too much stress works to create depression by causing over-activity of the body's stress response mechanism. It ignites hormones such as cortisol, the stress hormone, serotonin and dopamine, among others. These hormones have been linked to depression. When stress is sustained, it awakens an unhealthy level of these hormones that deviates them from their normal functions and causes depression. The situation is the same with the stress response. When difficult things happen to us, and we feel stressed, our stress response hormones come to our aid to help us cope. When the situation and the feelings that we go through pass, this stress response ought to reset. It ought to go back to its sterile state where it was inactive. When this does not happen, a susceptible person can experience depression.

When we lose anything at all, we may be at risk for depression, depending on the levels of stress that we experience from the loss. You can grieve after a loss, but for how long are you going to grieve? Its elongation and our inability to move on can lead to depression. When we lose a job and have to search for a new one for prolonged lengths of time, we can end up depressed. The state of being depressed can also cause other depressive episodes. You may feel that there is something wrong with you for you not to have gotten over the situation. Remarkably, you can effect changes to your body that relieves you of the stress that causes depression and anxiety by practicing self stimulation of your vagus nerve.

Can Our Lifestyle Affect The Stress and Depression or Anxiety Dynamic?

It is crucial to figure out if our lifestyle choices and emotional regulation are the factor that creates the link between stress and depression or anxiety. Can our lifestyle affect our response to stress? More importantly, can it affect it in a way that leads to depression and anxiety? There is undoubtedly a connection between stress and depression as there is between stress and anxiety. Also, that connection is complex, and it is impossible to dissect to a set of pointers. If we know that stress can cause depression and anxiety, the best course of action would be to prevent stress in the first place. The way to do this is to find out what causes stress.

Luckily, that is quite easy to spot. Stress has been linked to our lifestyle choices. It is what you are doing, what is going on in your life, and how you respond to each situation that often causes stress. In that case, stress can be minimized, prevented or eradicated if you make the right lifestyle choices. You may not have control over some of the occurrences, but you can make sure that you are not consciously causing the stress. People who undergo stress have forgotten how to take care of themselves. They have forgotten to look out for themselves, and they have allowed the circumstances in which they found themselves to overwhelm them. Getting rid of stress is, therefore, a conscious process. If you find that you have neglected exercise, you are smoking or drinking more than usual and engaging in substance abuse, you may want to rethink the consequences of your actions. You may want to begin to act in a way that puts your best interests ahead, and that makes positive lifestyle choices a priority.

Quoting Bruce McEwen, Ph.D., author of **The End of Stress as We Know It**, "Stress, or being stressed out, leads to behaviors and patterns that in turn can lead to a chronic stress burden and increase the risk of major depression." Many of the triggers for depression result in impairment of self-esteem. Let's consider a job loss: The reason that a job loss impacts us so much is that it results in the loss of social contacts and status in a way that we begin to feel bad about ourselves. This is even worsened when we are unable to replace the job as quickly as possible and when we get subjected to recruitment processes that feel demeaning. All of these can lead to depression. In the same manner, when we are expectant and unsure about a future occurrence, we become anxious. The stress that over thinking and ruminating over the many possibilities available for a situation is what leads to anxiety. Anxiety and depression therefore have a common root in stress. That stress is exactly what vagus nerve stimulation relieves.

Medical experts have pointed out that many of the changes that occur in the brain during depression are similar to those that occur during prolonged stress. Therefore, f you want to avoid or defeat depression, you should get rid of stress. If you want to reduce the anxiety in your life as well, you should lower the stressful activities in it. Limit your exposure to stress as much as possible. A great way to do this is by vagus nerve stimulation. The good news is that you no longer need to get surgery to do that. You can stimulate your vagus nerve from the comfort of your home. We will discuss vagus nerve stimulation exercises that you can engage to combat anxiety, stress and depression in chapter five of this book. Chapter six goes further to discuss metabolic processes that are aimed at stimulating your vagus nerve.

Treating Depression and Anxiety

While the treatment for stress might require calming effects, in some circumstances, treating anxiety and depression can go beyond that. Your doctor may put you through a combination of physical examination and screening tests to determine whether you have depression and anxiety. As with sharing some symptoms, depression and anxiety can use the same treatment methods. You may need to undergo therapy or to take medications to help ease your symptoms. You may be given an antidepressant, anti-anxiety medications and mood stabilizers. You may also have to go through cognitive behavioral therapy, interpersonal therapy or any other form of therapy that your doctor thinks is best for you. Make sure you let your doctor know before you try any alternative forms of therapy.

Preventing Anxiety, Stress, And Depression

Anxiety, stress, and depression are so common and life-altering that it is almost impulsive to want to avoid them. The Anxiety and Depression Association of America estimates that depression alone affects around fifteen million Americans every year. These three states come with so much discomfort that no one wants to be depressed, stressed, or anxious. Beyond that, they affect our bodies in profound ways. Preventing these conditions becomes a priority. However, of the three conditions, anxiety and depression are not seen medically as one of the conditions that you can consciously prevent. This is because spotting an exact cause for these conditions is often difficult. As for depression, you will usually not know that you are going through it or that you are about to experience it until it has happened. Some people are only able to identify their triggers after the first depressive episode.

You have to go through anxiety, stress and depression to know what ignited them, and you cannot prevent them without knowing what to guard against. It is possible to prevent depression from reoccurring if you have experienced an episode before. It is also easier to identify your triggers. You would have known which lifestyle changes can effectively work for you in preventing depression. You will also know which treatment works for you. In these cases, it may be possible to prevent depression. The situation is the same for both stress and anxiety. When you know that something stresses you, you can avoid that thing.

It is pivotal for you to put a lot of stress management techniques in place to help avoid anxiety and depression. You also have to make lifestyle changes that are tended toward prevention. Trying to position yourself in a way that you do not have depressive episodes or anxiety spasms has to do with identifying your triggers and avoiding them.

We have discussed some lifestyle changes below that can help you prevent anxiety, stress, and depression. If you do not want the disturbances that come with these mental states, you should integrate these lifestyle hacks into your everyday routine. Many of these tricks can transport your body into a state of calm by stimulating your vagus nerve.

SIMPLE HACKS TO MINIMIZE ANXIETY, STRESS, AND DEPRESSION

➢ Regular Exercise

Exercise is as great for your mind as it is for your body. It does a few things to your body that ease anxiety and depression. Exercising releases chemicals like endorphins that work to boost your mood. It reduces the chemicals that regulate your immune system that make anxiety and depression worse. Exercise can increase your body temperature, and by doing so, calm your central nervous system. If you want to get the best out of exercising, you should make it a routine. Exercising regularly can help treat anxiety and depression. If you need the inspiration to exercise more, join a team. Register with a gym and get moving. Physical activities can release mood-enhancing hormones that make your anxiety or depression better. Simple actions like walking can make you feel better. If you want to prevent anxiety and depression, make exercising a habit. Make sure that you always feel physically charged.

➢ **Minimize the Stress in your Life**

We have established that stress can trigger both anxiety and depression. If you are looking to feel better, you should work on reducing the stress in your life. What are those things that always stress you? What activities put an enormous amount of pressure on you? It is usually the case that we can do without many of those activities. Figure out where the stress is coming from and get rid of it. Although stress in its chronic form can cause depression and escalate anxiety, it is mostly avoidable. You are usually the one inflicting whatever is causing you stress, and you can eliminate it. You must only take on tasks that you can handle if you want to manage stress. Stop trying to prove your commitment to tasks that someone else can handle. Practice delegation. Practice mindfulness and meditate often. If something is beyond your control, let it go. Don't stay fixated on things you cannot control. Divert your energy to things that you can.

➢ Cut Out Social Media

While this may sound extreme, it is sometimes necessary. Social media puts us under the illusion that everyone's life is better than ours. If you think you cannot live without social media, reduce the time you spend on it. You would be surprised by the quality that your life can assume without social media in it. You will also be surprised by how much time you have been dedicating to social media. Cutting back on social media can quickly improve your life and open you up to a kind of mental clarity that you did not know you needed. What do you gain from hearing all about other people's lives? Mainly a sense that there is something wrong with yours. You do not need that.

Some practical tips for dealing with the social media bug in your life include deleting the apps from your phone, accessing social media from the web only, deciding to visit social media with a purpose and checking in with yourself to see that you are following this rule every time you log in. If you can handle it, delete your social media profiles altogether, but make sure you think it through before making the decision. Depression is usually propelled by a feeling of underachievement that causes low self-esteem, and social media is a pivotal trigger of that.

➢ Reduce the Choices You Have to Make

Organize your life in a way that you don't have to make choices each day. Decision making can be strenuous, and it can be exhausting to have to think so much. Researchers have found that having too many choices causes significant stress that is capable of leading to depression. Psychologist Barry Schwartz emphasized this in his book, **The Paradox of Choice,** where he stated that people who try to maximize their choices by working to choose the best from a list of alternatives face higher rates of depression. We all have choices to make, and we approach this differently. It is always best to simplify your life and your daily choices if you notice that deciding over which alternative works for you causes you stress. Practice fast decision making and do not reminisce over your choices. Decide over things as quickly as you can and avoid ruminating over whether you have made the right choice. If it is possible, delegate your decision making to somebody as capable as you are.

➤ Get Adequate Sleep

The National Sleep Foundation asserts that people with insomnia have a tenfold risk of developing depression when placed side by side with people who sleep well. Not only does sleep help your body to function well, but it also keeps your mind in proper shape. If you want to prevent depression from occurring, get adequate sleep. If you need help with sleeping, you can try keeping your phone away, ending TV and other screen time two hours before bedtime, meditating, and making your room sleep ready and cozy. These sleep routines can also help you to feel less anxious. Dark rooms tend to ignite sleep, so you may want to turn off the lights. Caffeine can keep you awake by making you active, so avoid taking it long before bedtime, advisably after noon.

➢ Maintain a Healthy Diet

A balanced diet can keep depression away in ways that you will never understand. For example, researchers have found that a high-fat diet can be equal to chronic stress in terms of the effects that it has on our body. Overeating fat can, therefore, cause depression. If you do not take the nutrients that you need, your body and mind will not be fortified against conditions such as depression and even anxiety. You can prevent depression and chronic anxiety by eating well. Make sure that your diet contains less sugar and fats and does not contain processed food. Include salmon and nuts into your diet to introduce Omega-3 fatty acids into what you eat. By eating well, you prepare yourself for the worse, and your body and mind can tackle conditions like depression and anxiety before they arise.

➤ Avoid Toxicity

We can become stressed by just listening to toxic people talk. If you have lots of people in your life that bring negativity with them and make everyday choices more difficult, dissociate from them. A 2012 study found that negative social interactions activated the release of higher levels of two proteins called cytokines, which are associated with depression. Toxic people can make us feel bad about ourselves and can lead us to develop lower self-esteem. If you discover that someone makes you feel bad about yourself, you should avoid that person. Avoid people that give you bad vibes. Are they carrying negative remarks about you within your circle? It may be time to detach from them and start creating associations that are beneficial for your physical and mental wellbeing. Develop friendships with people who respect you and who are willing to listen to your opinion. Look after your wellbeing by regulating your relationships. This way, you can keep your depression and anxiety triggers to a minimum. Besides, it has been found that laughing can activate your vagus nerve. Healthy social interactions can do the same too. If you always feel anxious or depressed, this might be all that you need to begin to live healthy. You cannot achieve that if all the people around you are toxic and negative.

➢ Look After Your Weight

Our weight is one of the most crucial triggers for low self-esteem. People who think they have excessive weight or not enough weight tend to feel bad about themselves. The Centers for Disease Control and Prevention points out that obesity can be linked to depression. Out of the forty-three percent who were found to be obese in a National Survey, a larger part of them were also depressed. If you want to prevent depression, you should maintain a healthy weight. You can do this by sleeping and eating well while maintaining your exercise schedule.

➢ Develop Great Relationships

Now that you have detached from toxic people, you should replace these people with people who uplift, motivate, and encourage you. Surround yourself with people who make you laugh. Develop a strong support system and work to ensure that your social life is great. If you have a great support network in place, you are more likely to push anxiety, depression and any other mental illness farther away.

➢ Stick to Your Treatment Plan

If you have experienced a depressive episode or anxiety spasms before, you already have a treatment regimen in place. If you want to avoid a reoccurrence, you have to follow this treatment routine and ensure that you take your prescribed medications. Experiencing successive depressive episodes is almost a given for people who have gone through the condition before. Anxious people may always be anxious too if they do not do anything about it. If you do not get adequate treatment, you propel a reoccurrence and you put your health in danger. Make sure that you are visiting your therapist as stipulated, for maintenance treatment. Follow your therapist's instructions and act on the coping mechanisms that he teaches you. You can avert a reoccurrence by not relapsing on your treatment plan.

➤ Take Note of the Side Effects of Your Prescription Medication

It is easy to take medications without any caution. If you want to avoid anxiety and depression, this shouldn't be the case. Many prescription medications have depression as a side effect. Read the label carefully before you take drugs. You can also let your doctor know and ask if you could get a different prescription. There could be other medications that can treat your condition as well, without the depression side effect. Some of the prescription medications that cause depression include birth control pills, corticosteroids, anticonvulsants, and so on. In some cases, medication may only increase your anxiety levels. If you're subject to anxiety and depression, it is important that you have an in-depth discussion with your doctor on what medication you should be taking.

➤ Get Adequate Treatment Where You Have Chronic Conditions

Chronic medical conditions can lead to depression. It is possible to manage such conditions in a way that they do not lead to depression. Let your doctor conduct a check up on you and determine which conditions you have. Make sure you follow the treatment plan that he recommends and always take the medications prescribed. Be sure to check that the medications themselves do not have depression as a side effect.

➤ Quit Smoking

Smoking is a trigger for depression and is generally extremely bad for your health. If you want to prevent depression, you must stop smoking and should slowly cut off nicotine of any kind. You may think that smoking calms you down in cases of anxiety but in reality, the nicotine contained in cigarette makes anxiety worse. It can escalate the symptoms, dampen your mood and mess with your brain. Motivate yourself to stop smoking by thinking about how much better your life will be after you quit. Prepare yourself for what is ahead and find people to keep you accountable.

➢ Quit Drinking

Like smoking, excessive drinking and substance abuse can lead to depression. If you continue to take alcohol after a depressive episode, you are also at risk of a reoccurrence. But that's not all. Alcohol is known to change the serotonin levels in the brain. It also upsets other neurotransmitters in the brain in a way that worsens anxiety. Although alcohol may make you feel better while you are taking it, when it wears off, you are likely to feel much worse. Reduce your alcohol intake and stop taking drugs. Set plans in place for how you will avoid alcohol in social situations. Drink more juice as it is healthier for you.

➢ Prepare Your Mind for Sad Events

There are anxiety and depression triggers that come with the normal tide of life, such as a death anniversary, a divorce, a job loss, and so on. Prepare ahead of time for how you would handle such situations if they occur in your life. If you have to be in a social gathering that is likely to trigger anxiety or depression, make up your mind on how you will handle the wave of sadness or uncertainty before you even get to experience it. You can go with someone to a burial, for example. Finding a way to cope is a pivotal step in preventing anxiety and depression.

Vagus nerve stimulation has been shown to improve anxiety, stress, and depression. It is a viable method of treatment for these three states. While vagus nerve stimulation can effectively ease treatment-resistant depression and anxiety, self-stimulation exercises go further to alleviate stress. We will discuss these self-stimulation exercises in chapter five of this book.

PART TWO

STIMULATING YOUR VAGUS NERVE

CHAPTER FOUR

VAGUS NERVE STIMULATION AS A NON-PHARMACOLOGICAL THERAPY

Although the mainstay of the treatment for individuals with nervous system-related disorder is pharmacological, non-drug treatments such as psychological interventions, the ketogenic diet and vagus nerve stimulation are also very suitable. Due to the high rate of risk involved in the treatment of nervous system related disorders, and the high cost of electrical stimulation of the vagus nerve, health practitioners have found various non-pharmacological means to cater for these disorders. These non-drug treatments have proven to be effective in managing varying degrees of seizure, heart diseases and nervous disorders. Of these non-pharmacological therapies, vagus nerve self-stimulation is the most widely recognized.

Over time, Vagus nerve self-stimulation has conveniently gained interest in the society. This may be attributed to the fact that it has continued to be effective and well tolerated in the management of several nervous system related abnormalities like vasovagal syncope, emotional dysregulation, low or abnormal heart rate variability, abnormal circadian rhythms, heart failures, cluster headaches, obesity, anxiety, stress and depression. Vagus nerve stimulation is reputably known to efficiently manage life threatening conditions like Alzheimer's disease, fibromyalgia, type 2 diabetes, seizure, arthritis, depression, cardiovascular disease, lung injury, traumatic brain injury, multiple sclerosis and some certain types of cancer.

Vagus nerve self-stimulation describes all the non-electrical and non-pharmacological techniques employed in increasing the vagal tone. It stresses the use of natural methods in stimulating the vagus nerve. Aside from the many benefits of vagus nerve self-stimulation, it can serve as a prophylactic therapy for always keeping the vagal tone in good shape. A decrease in vagal tone is implicated in the prognosis of a wide range of diseases. Vagal stimulation is the key to reset most pathophysiological states of the body resulting in a health improvement by reshaping neural networks. The biological pathway for vagal stimulation includes vagal reflexes and substantial and sustained impulses to the nucleus tractus solitarius. This is what the electrical impulses of vagus nerve stimulation mimic. This book offers you useful tools that have proven to stimulate the vagal pathway naturally, without the aid of electrical devices.

There are several options of non-pharmacological vagal nerve stimulation, including meditation, yoga, tai-chi, intermittent fasting and of course massages. Activities to focus on are breathing techniques, muscle stretching, consumption of specific food and beverages, facial immersion in cold water and praying among other things. Each of these non-pharmacological methods will be discussed in detail in the succeeding pages. Aside from the low-cost implication of vagus nerve self-stimulation, it can conveniently be performed at the comfort of your home. Interestingly, you don't necessarily need any special supervision to start your non-pharmacological vagus nerve self-stimulation therapy. What you will learn in the next pages of this guide is sufficient to begin your vagus nerve self-stimulation therapy.

Does Your Vagus Nerve Require A Stimulation?

There are numerous diseases associated with the vagus nerve. This is because the vagus nerve is a long nerve extending from the brain and passing behind the ear down through the neck into the trunk on both sides of the body, innervating several organs as it moves. This makes the vagus nerve prone to easy damage. If the vagus nerve becomes damaged, those organs it supplies will automatically be affected. Common symptoms of vagus nerve damage include:

- Pain in the ear

- Loss of gag reflex

- Trouble swallowing

- Difficulty in speaking or loss of voice

- A hoarse or wheezy voice

- Breathing abnormalities

- Unusual heart rate

- Abnormal blood pressure

- Decrease gastric acid production

- Abdominal bloat

- Abdominal pain

- Nausea or vomiting

- Incoordination

- Headaches

- Anxiety

- Depression

If you experience any of these symptoms, then you should consider a vagus nerve stimulation. However, the degree and occurrence of these symptoms depends on the part of the vagus nerve that has been affected. Prophylaxis self-stimulation of the the vagus nerve can help keep the vagus nerve and the entire nervous system under check. Therefore, whether or not your body displays signs of nervous system disorder, you should consider a vagus nerve self-stimulation.

CLINICAL APPLICATION OF VAGUS NERVE STIMULATION

There are hundreds of benefits of vagus nerve stimulation raging from the treatment of epilepsy to inflammation and treatment of medication-resistant depression. Vagus nerve stimulation is a potent drug-free alternative for managing several cases of persistent ill-health. Since the afferent vagus nerve transmits gut feelings of anxiety and fear to the brain, it is important to counter its effect to enhance adequate emotion regulation. The effectiveness of vagus nerve stimulation has been linked to high vagal tone. A high vagal tone index is expressed in a physical and psychological wellness. Low vagal tone index on the other hand is associated with inflammation, anxiety, depression, loneliness, negative moods, incoordination, heart attacks, and stroke. Studies have shown the clinical application of vagus nerve stimulation, some of which are discussed here.

Vagus Nerve In Treatment Of Epilepsy

Epilepsy affects 1% of the population and costs a lot of money to treat. Vagus nerve stimulation in the treatment of epilepsy was first used in the early 1880s by JL Corning who believed strongly that seizures were caused by changing the cerebral blood flow. By 1988, the first chronic implantable stimulator was adapted for treatment of drug-resistant epilepsy. This stimulator was approved by the FDA in 1997 to treat partial onset seizures that was nonresponsive to pharmacological control. The vagus nerve plays a role in quenching kindling of seizures in areas susceptible to heightened excitability including the limbic system, thalamus, and thalamocortical projections. Stimulating the vagus nerve therefore will help heighten this role. Vagus nerve stimulation may also affect structures in the midbrain and hindbrain which will facilitate seizure suppression. Vagus nerve stimulation increases activity in the locus coeruleus and the raphe nuclei. It also regulates the downstream release of norepinephrine and serotonin both of which have antiepileptic effects. Vagus nerve stimulation success in treating refractory epilepsy with few side effects provides for its rapid expansion to both additional conditions and to a wider population. Vagus nerve stimulation has long been adapted as a treatment for resistant epilepsy in pregnant women. Studies show that expecting mothers with epilepsy have high risk of mortality during delivery. However, as a non-pharmacological treatment, vagus nerve stimulation is beneficial for seizure control in pregnancy with no risk to the developing fetus.

Chronic epileptic seizures propose a substantial impact on children's neurodevelopmental and social outcome, as well as a lasting impact on their families. Children with epilepsy often experience psychiatric and cognitive difficulties. They also express poor social outcomes as adults. Antiepileptic medications have shown high profile side effects that adversely affect behavioral characteristics in susceptible children. Therefore, in children with easily controlled epilepsy, there is a high risk of psychological and psychiatric disturbance.

Children with absence epilepsy, benign rolandic epilepsy and autism have exhibited aggressive behavior, depression and anxiety. Several researches have gone into discovering the best method to effectively treat epilepsy in pediatric patients. Vagus nerve stimulators have been found to effectively treat pediatric epilepsy with minimal side effects. Although vagus nerve stimulation is only approve by the Food and Drug Administration in children above twelve years of age, children of 1 year in age and even neonates have benefited from the non-pharmacological therapy in controlling epilepsy.

Vagus Nerve Stimulation In Treatment Of Stress, Anxiety And Depression

Clinical and experimental studies indicate that stress and anxiety are closely associated with the elevation of the immune system resulting in increased production of pro-inflammatory cytokines. These circulating cytokines induce depression, thus lowering the vagal tone. This prolongs the symptoms expressed as low energy, low moods and lack of motivation. Anxiety and stress therefore, cause elevated levels of cytokine protein circulation in the blood stream, which may predispose one to depression. It would appear therefore that anxiety can lead to depression in the same way that stress does.

Your doctor may put you through a combination of physical examination and screening tests to determine whether you have depression and anxiety. Like some of the symptoms, depression and anxiety can use the same treatment methods. You may need to undergo therapy or take medications to help ease your symptoms. You may be given an antidepressant, anti-anxiety medications and mood stabilizers. You may also have to go through a cognitive behavioral therapy, interpersonal therapy or other forms of therapy that your doctor thinks are best for you. Nonetheless, increasing the vagal tone through a series of vagus nerve stimulation therapies has proven to conveniently treat depression, anxiety and stress. Stimulating the vagus nerve against depression is effective in both adults and children.

Vagus Nerve Stimulation In Treating Inflammatory Diseases

As discussed in chapter two, we have seen that vagus nerve stimulation is conveniently used as an anti-inflammatory treatment option. It has effectively managed the following inflammatory conditions:

Sepsis

Sepsis is typically resulting from a systemic bacterial infection and chronic activation of the pro-inflammatory cytokine cascade discussed in chapter two. Sepsis is estimated to be a multibillion dollar health care burden that cost $22, 000 per patient, and affects up to 18 million people every year. Several studies have gone into the management of sepsis using vagus nerve stimulation and have been proven effective with limited risk. Preventing inflammation in pediatric patients without the use of pharmaceuticals is vital because neonates, especially preterm infants, are mostly susceptible to developing sepsis since their immune system is still underdeveloped and susceptibility to perinatal infections like chorioamnionitis is high.

Vagus nerve stimulation regulates inflammation by modulating the cytokine cascade. Therefore substantial stimulation of the vagus nerve is an effective treatment of sepsis in both adults and infants.

Pain

Application of vagus nerve stimulation extends to widespread inflammatory disorders associated with chronic or intermittent bouts of pain such as fibromyalgia and migraines. Patients with fibromyalgia and depression have reported decreased sensation of pain after being treated with vagus nerve stimulation. Vagus nerve stimulation rapidly reliefs pain in patients with chronic pain ailment and migraine. Cluster headaches have successfully been treated by stimulating the vagus nerve at the neck region. Although more research and randomized trials are needed, vagus nerve stimulation remains the spring of hope for treating fibromyalgia and migraines.

Obesity

Although vagus nerve stimulation would not likely be recommended as a first-line defense against obesity, research has been conducted on the effects of vagus nerve stimulation on diet and weight. Researchers have tried to evaluate vagus nerve stimulation in relation to using it as an adjunct treatment in controlling obesity. Finding alternative treatments to obesity is vital considering that a large percentage of adults and adolescents in the United States are greatly overweight. Studies have shown that vagus nerve stimulation practices have significantly caused weight loss. Stimulating the vagus nerve results in attenuated hunger and food cravings. It also results in a decrease in intestinal caloric absorption since increase vagal tone can alter peptides that will change gut motility and absorption. The use of vagus nerve self-stimulation practices is an attractive means of controlling weight and managing obesity.

Cardiovascular Diseases

Vagus nerve stimulation has an impact on cardiovascular control due to the convergence of impulses in the autonomic control centers of the brain stem. The descending cardiac branch of the vagus nerve is vital for normal cardiac function. Atherosclerosis for example, which often predisposes affected patients to coronary heart diseases, is believed to be due to low-grade systemic inflammation. Remember that, because high vagal tone is a useful anti-inflammatory tool, vagus nerve stimulation is important in treating cardiac dysfunction and atherosclerosis. Stimulating the vagus nerve also provides a therapeutic application for preventing heart failure. Vagus nerve stimulation has been found to effectively modulate inflammatory functions in severe hypertension. There is a close relation between cardiovascular diseases, inflammation and vagal activity that can be improved by accurately stimulating the vagus nerve.

Lung Injury

Experiments have shown that several respiratory diseases can be managed with vagus nerve stimulation therapy. Vagus nerve stimulation is currently considered as a treatment for ventilator-induced lung injury due to pressure induced damage to the alveoli. Severe lung infection leads to inflammation which increases the likelihood of ventilator-induced lung injury. Several other respiratory disorders like acute respiratory distress syndrome and acute lung injury can escalate in sepsis and hence, pronounced pulmonary inflammation. Vagus nerve stimulation as said earlier remains a potent anti-inflammatory tool. Vagus nerve stimulation has been shown to treat gut and lung injury at the same time. It prevents intestinal barrier failure and protects against lung injury caused by several other diseases like hemorrhagic shock.

Stroke And Traumatic Brain Injury (TBI)

Stroke and traumatic brain injury are well known causes of widespread neural inflammation which can be alleviated by stimulating the vagus nerve. The anti-inflammatory properties of vagus nerve stimulation in cytokine upregulation and rebalancing of neurotransmitters released into circulation may provide a significant level of care to these patients and efficiently modulate injury due to trauma or ischemia.

Diabetes

Diabetes is another inflammatory-related disorder that also benefits from vagus nerve stimulation therapy.

Recent studies have shown the pathophysiology of diabetes and other related disorders. It is suggested that vagus nerve stimulation is useful in treating these disorders. Diabetes type 2 for instance, was shown to be a factor of increased risk for cardiovascular diseases. This fact was attributed to the sympathovagal imbalance resulting from these disorders.

Rheumatoid Arthritis

Rheumatoid arthritis is a chronic, inflammatory autoimmune disease which results in chronic synovial inflammation and damage to bone and cartilages due to release of cytokines and progressive inflammatory damage. The suppression of anti-inflammatory cholinergic pathways plays a critical role in rheumatoid arthritis. Vagal tone plays a great role in modulating rheumatoid arthritis. Vagus nerve stimulation is thus implicated in preventing rheumatoid arthritis.

CHAPTER FIVE

IMPROVING VAGAL TONE

The vagus nerve achieves total control over your joy through your vagal tone. Your vagal nerve and your parasympathetic nervous system are responsible for restoring your body to a state of rest after a shocking event passes. They work to balance the effect of adrenaline or the fight-or-flight response. This process is referred to as taking your body back to homeostasis. Your vagal tone is the measurement of your vagal response. Hence, everyone has a different vagal tone. Your vagal tone can be low or high. It could be elevated above the normal or depressed below normal. The vagal nerve achieves this state of calm by releasing a neurotransmitter called acetylcholine. In a nutshell, the vagus nerve is the driving force behind the parasympathetic nervous system. A low vagal tone can result in a wide range of health issues. When the vagal tone is high, the body will be in an increased state of calm. This is indicative of overall excellent health. The state of the vagal tone is influenced by several factors, including stress, genetics, anxiety, and so on.

While the functioning of the vagal nerve is biological, this is not often the case today. The increased number of stressors in our daily lives has changed the way our bodies react to emergencies. It would seem that instead of having a significant event that requires our fight-or-flight response, what we have is an increased number of small stressful situations that are happening rather fast. Very often, our body is not able to get back to normal homeostasis. Our entire nervous system seems displaced and highly detached from its biological function. While the body is trying to relax from a stressful situation, another one usually happens in quick succession that makes getting back to calm almost impossible. It would appear that in today's digital world, our bodies remain in a perpetual state of alarm. As a result of this, it is essential to learn how to improve your vagal tone. There are several ways to intervene in this displacement of our normal body functioning to create the calm needed with each daily stressor. As you go from one alarming event to another during your day, you should be conscious of how to return your body to a more relaxed state.

Now that you know how vital the vagus nerve is to your wellbeing, why don't you take charge of your mind, body, and soul by controlling the vagal switch? You can turn it on when environmental circumstances depress it. You can switch it up or better still, choose to leave it in a constant stable and elevated state. Achieving this is simpler than you imagine. To control the vagus nerve, you must put the vagal tone under check. Improving your vagal tone gives you total control of your vagus nerve. There are numerous ways to boycott the famous electrical stimulation of the vagus nerve and still improve your vagal tone. We speak of vagus nerve stimulation by introducing simple health practices to your daily activities.

In this chapter, we will be showing you practical methods of reducing the alarming effect of environmental impulses on your body. You will learn the various techniques for improving your vagal tone through simple exercises.

Vagus Nerve Stimulation Exercises

Stimulating the vagus nerve can make us instantly happy. This makes it an essential part of nervous system regulation. You can initiate healing for a variety of mental health problems like anxiety and depression by stimulating the vagus nerve. While there is a pharmacological therapy for stimulating the vagus nerve, there are also methods that do not involve surgery and other pharmacological processes and which can be performed safely at home. These are the vagus nerve self-stimulation exercises. Remember that your vagus nerve passes through several parts of your body. That indicates that you can stimulate it from any of these places. The following exercises can help you unlock the power of your vagus nerve within minutes.

Humming

You can improve your vagal tone because the vagus nerve passes through the inner ear and the vocal cords. When you hum, the vibration gets to these places, and so it induces your vagus nerve, causing an increased vagal tone. All you have to do is pick your favorite song and hum the tune. You will feel great in an instant.

Controlled Breathing

This is a method of breathing that focuses on moving your belly and diaphragm while you breathe. It is one of the fastest ways to stimulate your vagus nerve and induce your entire nervous system to an elevated state. Make sure that you slow down your breathing as this is what would stimulate your vagus nerve. Our typical breathing speed is 10-14 breaths per minute, but when we slow this down to 5-7 breaths, we influence our vagus nerve to calmness. To achieve this calming effect of your breathing, count up to 5 when you inhale, hold the breath briefly and then exhale while you count to 10.

Valsalva Maneuver

This is another breathing technique that stimulates the vagus nerve. All you have to do is exhale through an almost closed airway. You achieve the effect by pinching your nose while you breathe with your mouth closed. Doing this improves your vagal tone by creating more pressure in your chest cavity.

Diving Reflex

This is one of the fastest ways to stimulate your vagus nerve. The diving reflex technique is carried out by splashing cold water on your face. Allow the water to go all the way from your scalp line to your lips. If this seems a little difficult to achieve, you can go for the alternative method of achieving the diving reflex, which includes holding some ice cubes against your face by putting the ice in a zip-lock bag. When the ice touches your face, you should hold your breath briefly. This vagus nerve stimulation method has the effect of slowing your heart rate, increasing the flow of blood to your brain, and relaxing your body.

A third method of achieving the diving reflex is by holding lukewarm water in your mouth and allowing the water to cover your tongue. Try to sense the water with your tongue. This can quickly relax you.

Stay Connected

Sometimes, all you need to stimulate your vagus nerve is a warm hug from someone you love. Well, your nerves would still be stimulated if you do not love them. Human connection can improve your vagal tone. This connection needs to be physical, though. Talking over the phone, text messaging and social media will definitely not help you improve your vagal tone. Great relationships can relax both your body and your mind. If you are accustomed to being alone, find ways to stay connected with other people even if this connection is only partial.

Gargling

This is similar to submerging your tongue in water. Put some water in your mouth and gargle as hard as you can. When you start to feel tears in your eyes, you have stimulated your vagus nerve using this method.

Laughing

Laughter can improve your vagal tone. It does this by releasing neurotransmitters that ease your vagal nerve.

Try to laugh when you feel stressed and laugh often to keep your vagus nerve in an elevated state.

Singing

Singing is one of the hobbies that may be good for your vagus nerve. If you love singing, that is a plus. If you don't, you should start now. You don't have to be a great singer. You just need to make sure you are doing it at the top of your lungs. Singing relaxes the muscles in the back of your throat and stimulates your vagus nerve by doing so.

Get a Massage

Massages are great for relaxing your vagus nerve. Whether you are massaging your feet, your neck or receiving a pressure massage, this exercise can stimulate your vagus nerve and go further to help reduce seizures and lower your heart rate and blood pressure. Massages stimulate your lymphatics, which in turn improves your vagal tone. So, go get a massage right now.

Take Cold Showers

Cold showers are great for improving your vagal tone. They may be uncomfortable at first, but as your body adjusts to the cold, you begin to feel relaxed. Your vagus nerve is activated, and you enjoy a calming effect. This is great especially during cold summer days.

Exercise Regularly

Exercise can stimulate the vagus nerve by inducing gut flow and gastric mobility. It doesn't have to be a tough exercise, though. Mild exercises can achieve this effect. Therefore, when you feel in low spirits, you can jog a couple of miles and you will feel an almost instant relief.

Yoga

Yoga is an excellent exercise for stimulating the vagus nerve. Yoga involves breathing and movement that helps digestion and blood flow, thereby increasing GABA (Gamma-aminobutyric Acid) levels. An increased GABA level is known to improve vagal tone as GABA itself is a calming neurotransmitter in the brain. In a related study, participants of a 12-week yoga course exhibited bigger changes in mood compared to their counterparts who engaged in walking exercises. Yoga has been proven to reduce anxiety levels as well and was found to alert the vagus nerve and make the participants feel better. If your vagus nerve is depressed, yoga may be what you need.

Meditation

Meditation is a great way to stimulate your vagus nerve. It does this by increasing your parasympathetic activity and sending calming sensations throughout your body. By practicing meditation and focusing your mind, you aid the release of neurotransmitters in the brain and increase your vagal tone. You also reduce your sympathetic activity and force your body to relax.

Tai Chi

Tai chi increases the activity in your parasympathetic nervous system and by doing so it enhances your vagal modulation. Yoga and tai chi have very similar effects on the vagus nerve and embody a calming sensation that quickly makes you feel better.

CHAPTER SIX

METABOLIC PROCESSES FOR IMPROVING VAGAL TONE

Aside from vagus nerve stimulation exercises, a great diet can improve your vagal tone. You already know that maintaining a balanced diet is critical to good health. To experience the calming effects of the vagus nerve, you should know how to improve your vagal tone using the body's metabolic activity.

In this chapter, we will discuss specific food cultures that can enhance your vagal tone. This includes supplements and eating methods that substantially stimulate your vagus nerve.

PROBIOTICS

Researchers have linked the health effects of gut bacteria to the vagus nerve. Gut bacteria improves brain function not only by reaching the brain itself but by enhancing vagal tone. One study showed that the probiotic Lactobacillus Rhamnosus improved GABA receptors in a controlled group of animals. This led to a reduction in the hormones causing anxiety, stress and depression. The behavior of the animals in the study was found to have improved greatly. The researchers were able to link the change in behavior and calm that the animals experienced to an enhanced vagal tone ignited by the gut-brain connection and the influence of the probiotic on them.

The same research was conducted on mice but in this case, the probiotic was removed. The results showed continued exhibition of anxiety, stress and depression. This confirms that the probiotic in question was responsible for making the animals feel better. When another probiotic, Bifidobacterium Longum, was introduced, the mice exhibited reduced levels of anxiety. The probiotics was found to have acted through the vagus nerve.

It would appear therefore that probiotics act to enhance vagal tone by increasing good bacteria in the gut.

OMEGA-3 FATTY ACIDS

Omega-3 fatty acids are essential to the proper functioning of your brain and your nervous system. However, your body cannot produce fatty acids by itself. These fatty acids help with the electrical impulses of your brain. Omega-3 fatty acids can help repair leaky guts, can improve mental health and as it has been found out recently, can increase vagal tone.

This special type of fats does this by increasing heart rate variability and lowering the heart rate. Both activities can stimulate the vagus nerve. Omega-3 fatty acids are primarily gotten from fish (for example salmon) and nuts, and are known to enhance parasympathetic activity. If you want to improve your vagal tone, you can try eating lots of omega-3 rich foods.

INTERMINENT FASTING AND VAGAL TONE

Another important vagus nerve stimulation method that requires in-depth discussion in this book is intermittent fasting. It would appear that vagus nerve self-stimulation has found a place in our weight loss efforts. This has been made possible through the now popular concept of intermittent fasting. You can now lose weight and enjoy the calming effects of an elevated vagus nerve at the same time. To understand how intermittent fasting influences vagus nerve self-stimulation, we have to first understand what the concept itself means. This chapter will take you through knowing what intermittent fasting is about, why there is a crave for it, and how it can improve your vagal tone.

Understanding Intermittent Fasting

Our body image culture is taking a new dimension. Different methods for the successful approach and execution of a glamorous body spring up regularly. This set of principles is taking over the beauty, health, and wellness industry, especially the weight loss propositions that state how we all should look. The latest is the concept called intermittent fasting. It has been shown by one study after the other to be entirely or at least to no small extent a healthy practive. Intermittent fasting carries enormous promises of making our health and weight loss goals come true. But it does more than this: intermittent fasting is apparently good for the brain too. A lot of people wonder how a fast can do all that. And for good reasons. Perhaps, understanding what intermittent fasting is can help you see how it can improve overall health.

Intermittent fasting is not a diet. It is instead an eating pattern that emphasizes control over our eating periods and, in no time, the autonomic system. It stipulates that we should adjust the times when we eat in a way that we give our bodies a break as often as possible. Intermittent fasting suggests that we can maintain our regular eating schedule in a nutrition sense but then restrict our feeding within the specified time window. This leaves us with the times when we are not eating. This time is our fasting window. Proponents of the concept have tried to make fasting easy by incorporating short term fasts into our regular daily or weekly routine. Thus, we have days or weeks when we can eat all the food we want within a specified interval and embark on a fast within the rest of the period on our hands. While this may be good for some people and bad for others, intermittent fasting principles have envisaged the possible obstacles and have sorted these out accordingly. Thus, there are different types of intermittent fasting from which you can choose. You can go through them and select which one best suits you and your lifestyle. Some of the methods are so easy to carry out that they flow effortlessly into your everyday routine. In this way, intermittent fasting affords everyone the possibility of undertaking it, therefore accessing its benefits the body and, of course, vagal tone. It is advisable to begin with the intermittent fasting methods that you find yourself comfortable with, and then build your way up to some of the other, more advanced, methods.

Vagal nerve dysfunction typically arises from a low vagal tone manifestation. Stimulating the vagus nerve can appropriately take care of this condition. Since the treatment of vagal tone represent lifestyle changes, which intermittent fasting is part of, it is safe to include intermittent fasting practice in the management of vagal tone.

WHAT IS INTERMITTENT FASTING?

Fasting is a state that we all partake in whether or not we are conscious about it. When we are asleep, our bodies are in a state of fast. Intermittent fasting is about recognizing the benefits and integrating them into our everyday life with some conscious efforts. The concept of intermittent fasting does not necessarily have religious connotations. It is instead a way to key into the benefits that abound in abstaining from food for our overall health and fitness. Fasting started as a medical practice to enable the body to heal itself. It is one of the oldest therapies for healing and prevention, and it continues to be recommended by doctors. According to Paracelsus, fasting is the most excellent remedy. It was popular in ancient Greece and has been handed down to us. Fasting was also considered as a tradition and was used to fulfill certain customs in the past. Fasting also has a religious connotation today.

Intermittent fasting, on the other hand, is a recent development. People are no longer skipping meals to fulfill religious or cultural rites. They are not going without food as a method for ensuring the healing and prevention of illness. People are now consciously scheduling their meals to certain times of the day or week so that at the other times, the body is left without food and is able to get rid of impurities using its natural processes. Often people do this to enable them to lose excess fat. However, intermittent fasting does not qualify as a diet or even a specific weight loss strategy because it is almost effortless.

Intermittent fasting is an eating pattern in which you move between periods of eating and fasting. The concept is not much concerned about the foods that you are eating within this period, as it is with when you eat them. Thus, intermittent fasting takes you through a schedule of eating and fasting. The methods are varied, and each one specifies how you perform the split. You can choose to go for the day method or the week method. In the former case, the periods of eating and fasting are divided between the hours of the day, while in the latter case, the split occurs between days of the week. There are a lot of intermittent fasting methods, but every one of them is classified into these two broad divisions. You either choose to go for the daily splits of when to eat or the weekly splits. The critical thing to be aware of when you are carrying out intermittent fasting is that you are going through a cycle. This cycle is one in which you eat sometimes, and you abstain from eating at other times.

Intermittent fasting is, therefore, a somewhat simplified concept. You can get into an intermittent fast by merely extending the fast that occurs every night. Some people are already doing this by their lifestyle but do not even know. Once you skip breakfast, you might be on an intermittent fast without even knowing. In more specific terms, if you want to try this method of intermittent fasting, all you have to do is skip breakfast and take your first meal at noon while taking dinner at 8 pm. That 8 pm meal should be your last for the day. By doing this, you are fasting for sixteen hours while eating for eight. This is the most popular method of intermittent fasting, and it is called the 16/8 method.

Intermittent fasting is about the time-division between eating and fasting.

At first, your body might find intermittent fasting discomforting, but as time passes, you will find that it renews your energy levels. You may have to battle hunger when you are starting, but like other forms of fasting, it only gets better. While you can eat during the specified period, you can only take liquid substances like water and coffee during the time apportioned for fasting. You can take supplements during intermittent fasting also. However, you cannot take beverages that are high in calories during your fasting window. You can only take drinks with low calories, like homemade fruit juice, tea or coffee that do not have extra condiments. Intermittent fasting is, therefore, basically about scheduling your meal plans in a way that certain aspects of the day or the week go without food. It is a catch-all term for "time-restricted eating" within which you eat only during a specific time window.

Aaron Zimmerman

HOW OUR MODERN DIET IS A PROBLEM

With the rise in health hazards, it is becoming increasingly necessary to question the safety promise of the modern diet. Health conditions such as obesity, diabetes, heart failures, and so on are on the rise. While doctors and other health practitioners often point us to the medical cure for the disease, it would be worthwhile if we looked into the root cause of such conditions. Isn't there something that we are not doing right that is making us sick in the first place? Why have the various dieting methods not curbed the situation? The persistence of health troubles only shows that there is a foundational problem. Perhaps, it is what we put into our bodies that causes all the negativity that we have to encounter and handle.

We need to take another look at what we are eating. Our food choices have changed in a few decades, and it appears that lifestyle changes are also affecting the choice of what we eat. The procedure that food goes through to get into our plates is the primary cause of the diet problem that we have to deal with today. We now focus on processed food. But is this kind of diet perfect for us? I think the answer is in the statistics: about 78.6 million people in the United States are reportedly obese, and with obesity come a lot of other health concerns that these people have to handle.

Virtually all that we eat today is processed in a way or another. Even the food items you buy when you choose to cook your meals yourself have gone through one chemical change or the other before getting to you. The effects are visible when we continually feed these into our bodies. It is like taking poison. The modern diet is laced with additives, sugar, and chemicals. It would appear, therefore, that the nutrients in our food come to us differently. They are no longer whole when we consume them. We take in nutrients that have been diminished in value, and our bodies absorb them in their reduced state. It seems that some of us have chosen this life of unhealthiness. We consume extra sugar despite the depleted nature of the food that we eat. We then continually find ways to correct the situation. We do not want the extra weight or the health consequences of taking low-quality food and more sugar. Our numerous diet plans seem futile. Something needs to change.

In the last two decades, dieting has risen quickly to correct the situation. However, the problem with dieting is that you have to let go of some nutrients while you are working on keeping others. This results in a situation where your body has to make due with the limited nutrients that it gets from your diet. Whether we are dieting or not, there is something inherently wrong with the modern diet. We have realized this, and we are trying so hard to change this in a lot of wrong ways. We are eating additives, sugar, processed fats, and other unhealthy food. The problem is that because most of our food items are processed, we get to eat these additives regardless of whether we are making the food ourselves or not. Now, we want to correct that. This situation makes it critical that we become concerned about our diets and find our way back to what is substantially healthy for us.

SCIENCE BEHIND INTERMITTENT FASTING

Our body lives on energy. We need certain levels of energy to sustain us. This is the case whether or not we are in a fast. The primary source of energy for our bodies is glucose, and it is gotten from carbohydrates. The glucose passes through the liver and the muscles to our bloodstream to keep us active. Any glucose that is not in use is often stored in the liver and muscles. When we steer clear of providing our bodies with nutrients in a fast, we deny our bodies of glucose. For the period of the fast, the body will use up the glucose that is stored away. This happens within eight hours of not eating and transports the body to a state known as gluconeogenesis. Studies show that during gluconeogenesis, there is a heightened calory burn. The body burns the fats previously-stored into glucose to create the energy that it needs. However, the fat will run out in the end. When it does, the body moves into starvation and begins to burn body tissues. This extreme stage of metabolism takes place after twenty-four hours. Hence, it is considered safe to stay without food for twenty-four hours where no medical conditions are negating the possibility to do so. This is why intermittent fasting is possible. Staying without food for sixteen hours or less in a day will burn all the fat stored but will not translate into starvation.

Additionally, intermittent fasting is good for our mitochondria. It causes it to stay fused, and in the process, we are more active and full of energy. This also affects our memory positively and acts as an additional anti-aging mechanism.

WHY YOU WANNA FAST

The word fasting does not sound that inviting. Even though people skip meals or follow a strict diet to enable them to lose weight, they cringe when they hear the word "fast." Intermittent fasting then feels like just a branded type of fasting. This new way to fast is a somewhat effective weight loss strategy. In spite of this ability to burn fats that the concept possesses, it is not a diet. It is just a strategy for conditioning your mind to skip meals at certain times in a day or on certain days in a week. It is about preparing your body for eating at alternate intervals. In this wise, intermittent fasting is just a pattern of eating. Remember that you formed the habit of eating three meals a day. Intermittent fasting proponents are saying that you should rearrange the order in which you eat. In other words, form new habits that let you eat at different and more efficient intervals. Additionally, you should dedicate the time within which you are not eating to avoiding high volumes of calories. Intermittent fasting is, therefore, merely the discipline to schedule your meals or to reschedule them as the case may be.

Intermittent fasting does not tell you what to eat. You are not required to change what you are eating. You do not have to reduce fats, take more proteins, or follow any of the other common rules of dieting. All you need to do is to set the time when you will take your meals every day and then follow through on it. Intermittent fasting is, therefore, about changing when you are eating. But why would anyone want to do that?

To give a simplistic response to the question above it is sufficient to say that it is worthwhile to undertake intermittent fasting: aside from putting your weight worries to rest, it causes heart rate variability to surge and it promotes a decline in metabolism. Both events are a definite trigger for vagus nerve functioning. With intermittent fasting, you do not necessarily have to miss out on calories if you love them. All you have to do is integrate a fast into your everyday life. Your calories can stay the same, and you still get to lose unnecessary fat from all your viscera without even noticing. Thus, promoting effective parasympathetic innervation through your vagus nerve. Your vagal tone is elevated, and you will experience much less cardiac malfunctions, normal blood pressure elevation, and the relieving effects of sympathetic innervation. You become more relaxed and able to handle life's troubles better.

Intermittent fasting is known to help you build muscle mass more healthily. Thus, you will get the kind of weight loss that leaves you active. You may look lean when you use intermittent fasting, but you will not be fragile. Intermittent fasting is, therefore, a great way to build muscle without hitting the gym. If you want to wear off unnecessary fat from your viscera, lose weight healthily, and improve your vagal tone, intermittent fasting is one of the healthiest options you have got. Most people are likely to be committed to the process because all that you have to do is stick to a schedule for eating. Once this becomes a pattern, you will start seeing visible results. People love the concept as a weight loss and fitness strategy because it can be executed with ease. You may want to fast for the same reasons too.

BENEFITS OF FASTING

Fasting of any kind, despite its initial discomfort, comes with lots of benefits.

Scientists are performing sample fasts on animals to find out whether the concept of intermittent fasting is healthy or not. Some research has been held in the past, and other are still underway. In one study, researchers compared intermittent fasting and dieting over one year and found that the impact of the two on weight loss was the same. They also found that the two concepts had similar impacts on other health conditions, like heart rate and blood pressure. In a similar study, researchers found that intermittent fasting could lower the risk of type 2 diabetes. As we have discussed above, for intermittent fasting to be able to do any of these things, it would have to carry the body through a process. There must be some internal functions that the fasting method performs within our bodies. Experts have found that the effects of intermittent fasting may go beyond affecting only our bodies, though. These wide-ranged benefits associated with intermittent fasting are what we are going to discuss in this section of the book. Let us take a look at some of the ways that intermittent fasting goes beyond adjusting our bodies to affecting other areas of our lives positively.

MENTAL BENEFITS OF INTERMITTENT FASTING

Researchers have found that intermittent fasting carries some benefits for our mental health. Some findings show that intermittent fasting can increase mental clarity while boosting productivity. In a 2013 study, researchers found while using mice to undertake their study, that intermittent fasting can improve cognitive functions and brain structures. The researchers exposed a group of mice to food while keeping another group on intermittent fasting. The latter group exhibited better learning and memory than the former. Intermittent fasting thus improved the cognitive ability of the mice. It has had the same effects as humans. In this manner, intermittent fasting is excellent for improving mental health and memory. It sharpens the learning and retention ability of the brain in a way that enhances its memorization capacity and capability.

Another benefit of intermittent fasting is that it improves neuroplasticity. It does this by fighting inflammation. The effects that intermittent fasting has on the brain also make it possible for the brain to stay renewed instead of aging. This is possible because intermittent fasting induces anti-aging hormones. These added effects of intermittent fasting also result in increased learning abilities and better retention. Fasting goes further to boost the chances of recovery from significant hazards that would otherwise have been detrimental to the proper functioning of the brain. This eating method can help the brain heal quickly from any injury and lower the risk of neurodegenerative diseases such as dementia, Parkinson's disease, stroke and so on.

HEALTH BENEFITS OF INTERMITTENT FASTING

The health benefits of intermittent fasting are wide-ranged. There are a lot of health hazards that intermittent fasting can repair. However, intermittent fasting also works to improve the quality of our health, even if we were doing okay in that department. Intermittent fasting quickly adjusts weight issues. It is a rather convenient weight loss strategy. When you schedule your time window for eating, you position your body to burn all unwanted fat and thus keep you in shape. Intermittent fasting pushes the body into a metabolic state that burns off any excess fat. For people who are obese, intermittent fasting is rewarding. By burning off fat and bringing weight loss to reality, it also affords them an escape route from the hazards associated with obesity. Some studies have even hinted at a reduced risk of cancer for people who are on intermittent fasting. Although the study was conducted on animals, the positive effects for reducing cancer that the eating schedule is linked with have been suggested to result from its weight loss potential. Intermittent fasting is thus suitable for treating obesity and cancer by naturally shedding off the weight. Perhaps, the potential for reducing cancer that researchers hint at can also be traced to other factors such as a reduction in insulin levels and inflammation.

Other studies have found that intermittent fasting can reduce the risk of having heart disease and type 2 diabetes. Intermittent fasting can take care of the heart by getting rid of a fat known as triglycerides. Once the fat burning process takes this fat out of the body, the risk for heart disease is immediately removed. Intermittent fasting is known to improve health generally. For people who love to keep fit, intermittent fasting is excellent for building muscle mass. When people first begin to indulge the eating pattern, they are surprised at what it does for their bodies. They find that despite missing out on the gym and eating lots of food, they stay in great shape. Intermittent fasting can work on your muscles and reduce the necessity of both gyms and diet plans. Most people get into intermittent fasting for the weight loss benefits, but then, they are usually astounded by what it does in terms of building their muscle mass. About health, intermittent fasting can do wonders to keep you intact.

HOW INTERMITTENT FASTING IMPROVES OUR QUALITY OF LIFE

Several studies of different animals, including rodents, nematodes, and fruit flies, have shown that reducing calorie consumption by thirty to forty percent can extend life span. Similar studies have suggested that in some species of monkeys, eating less elongated their life span. The studies relating to the effect of consuming less in humans is at the moment, inconclusive. However, it is agreed that the reduction of calorie consumption in humans and the general intake of less food reduces the risks of various diseases, thereby elongating life. Eating fewer offsets the risk of certain diseases that are common in old age. Eating less food provides an avenue to increase periods in one's life when good health is abundant. We can easily make this healthy part of our lives a rather large portion by engaging intermittent fasting. While it is easy to want to stay healthy and have a high quality of life, it is difficult to eat less when we are hungry. Intermittent fasting provides a way to get around this. The concept does not tell you to reduce the quantity of food that you eat. Instead, by skipping your meals at certain times of the day, you will automatically reduce what you eat. In this way, intermittent fasting can deliver to you all the benefits associated with eating less. The periods of fasting will automatically translate into the less calorie consumption that you need for a healthy life.

Intermittent fasting thus improves our health. With the weight loss accruing also comes a level of fitness that is sought after. Eating and fasting within a consistent pattern can improve our quality of life by keeping us healthy and fit. It has been found that intermittent fasting has the capacity to prolong our lifespan.

BEHAVIORAL IMPROVEMENTS WITH INTERMITTENT FASTING

Intermittent fasting is known to improve behavioral patterns. A group of researchers found that intermittent fasting helped to improve body image in people with obesity. When people maintain the fast for a consistent period of eight weeks, they were less likely to engage in detrimental behavior like binge eating. Intermittent fasting was also found by the same study to reduce depression. Thus, the concept of controlled eating patterns had both psychological and behavioral effects on people who practiced. When you regulate when you eat, you eat less without putting any effort into the process. For instance, if you take your first meal at noon, you would have prevented yourself from overeating in the early hours of the morning. This automatically gets rid of any binge eating tendencies that you may have, especially when you are taking your last meal at 8 pm. Also, intermittent fasting has a way of conditioning your mind to eat precisely what your body needs. The fact of skipping some meals using your fasting periods quickly negates the fact of overeating. In this way, intermittent fasting helps you adjust your eating patterns without much effort on your part.

As a study in the Journal of Molecular Psychiatry found, intermittent fasting can activate the hunger hormone called Ghrelin and drive people into an elevated mood. The hormone is a natural antidepressant. During fasting, high levels of this hormone are activated, and its effects make people less depressed. Additionally, intermittent fasting can improve mood by removing the factors that would have caused the depression in the first place. Such factors include excessive weight gain. Intermittent fasting is regarded as the best weight loss strategy. When obese people lose weight, they tend to experience an elevated mood and also stay psychologically healthy.

INTERMITTENT FASTING HAS SOME EFFECTS ON OUR TIME AND MONEY

The fact of not eating within specified periods automatically saves us money. We spend less when we eat less. We can save up on food since what we buy lasts longer. Grocery shopping would then be a less regular activity, thereby saving your time in the process. Intermittent fasting can save you the time you spend cooking as well. These two benefits are among the very best reasons to try the eating pattern. If you want to keep more of your money or you want to spend less time on cooking, grocery shopping, and other food-related activities, you should try intermittent fasting. The concept will help you lose fat and save money doing so. Unlike the prevalent dieting methods, you will be missing the precise nutrient type that adds up to weight gain. Thus, your weight loss will be healthy. It won't be the type that crops up before you know it, and you don't have to spend lots of money or time achieving this.

INTERMITTENT FASTING CAN DIRECTLY IMPACT ON YOUR PERSONAL GROWTH

With the benefits that accrue from intermittent fasting in terms of psychological, behavioral, and health patterns, intermittent fasting frees you up to be able to pursue your personal growth goals. It leaves you with the time, the money, and the health conditions that make pursuing self-development possible. If these issues bedevil you, you may never remember to talk more about pursuing self-improvement. In this case, taking care of your body by providing it with the conditions in which it can perform great, rewards you with the ability and the time needed to pursue other worthy goals. Instead of going down the tunnel of depression that overeating can take you, you are on the opposite route. For people who are on different weight-loss strategies and not getting the results that they anticipate, intermittent fasting will accellerate their progress. When you take care of foundational issues like this, you have the time and the resources that you need to invest in growing yourself in other areas. Achieving this is what intermittent fasting is about

INTERMITTENT FASTING AS A NON-PHARMACOLOGICAL THERAPY FOR THE STIMULATION OF THE VAGUS NERVE

Intermittent fasting stimulates the vagus nerve by default. When you are fasting, you are allowing your digestive system to rest. This state of rest is what the vagus nerve aims to achieve. Whether you are abstaining from food completely or you are taking fewer snacks than you usually do, intermittent fasting improves parasympathetic activity and by doing so enhances your vagal tone. Intermittent fasting also increases your heart rate variability and by so doing positively affects parasympathetic activity and vagal tone.

Intermittent fasting is easy to implement and you could start fasting by merely postponing breakfast until noon. When you are eating your meals within an 8 hour window, you are already fasting and stimulating your vagus nerve without much effort.

Self stimulation of your vagus nerve is as much about the metabolic processes that you allow your body go through as it is about the exercises aimed at calming you down. While we have explored the exercises that can improve your vagal tone in an earlier chapter, we have seen three major metabolic methods for vagus nerve stimulation right here in this chapter. If you are feeling really stressed right now, you can try any of these methods to make you feel better. What's more? You can even make some of them a constant state for your body. For example, you can eat fish as much as possible and maintain an exercise schedule that you actually follow. The results of activating these practices are phenomenal.

CONCLUSION

Vagus nerve stimulation has proven to be a useful treatment tool for several diseases. It has been used to effectively treat seizures, depression, pain, anxiety, stroke, septicemia, and a wide variety of disease conditions. The importance of vagus nerve stimulation to cater for different classes of patients cannot be relegated. Several pieces of evidence have shown that vagus nerve stimulation can help quell inflammation in several autonomic and inflammatory disorders. This makes it useful for a broader range of patients, including ones in pediatric age.

Studies are continually going on to provide evidence of vagus nerve stimulation for several other conditions. Preliminary research has shown the effectiveness of vagus nerve stimulation on stroke, obesity, autoimmune diseases, and pain management, heart, and lung failures. Further studies are, however, needed to fully elucidate the mechanism of action that proves the vagus nerve stimulation potential in managing these disorders.

This book has shown the pathways through which vagus nerve exercises its actions. Nonetheless, a detailed pathway analysis that would focus on the mechanisms by which vagus nerve alters autonomic tone is essential to provide a further understanding of vagus nerve modification. We have seen how the vagus nerve interacts with the body's immune system to modify inflammatory tone by altering the release of pro-inflammatory and anti-inflammatory cytokines. Some of these key inflammatory markers have been duly summarized for you in chapter two. There is overwhelming evidence that proves that the vagus nerve is a vital component of the immune system, and manipulating the vagal tone is a profitable way to modulate the immune system. The use of vagus nerve self-stimulation in shaping vagal tone provides an exciting new opportunity for noninvasive therapeutic intervention in both adults and children.

Highlighted in this book are the various techniques needed for a successful vagus nerve stimulation. This book is an eye-opener to the various benefits of vagus nerve stimulation on our health and social environment. We have seen that even though vagus nerve stimulation proposes minimal risk to the patient, the benefits are much higher. In the event to avert the risk of electrical vagus nerve stimulation, a much milder form of stimulating the vagus nerve was found. This is what is virally known as vagus nerve self-stimulation. It promises to help you find fulfillment in life. It achieves this with the same mechanism as vagus nerve stimulation. The magnitude of impulses sent to the brain is what determines the level of stimulation. In order to effectively stimulate the vagus nerve, your body requires a substantial amount of impulses maintained at a constant rate. This is how the vagal tone gets increased. The various exercises covered in different sections of this book, if appropriately performed, will help you target the cause of your low vagal tone and revitalize it. Vagus nerve self-stimulation can be used as a prophylactic therapy to prevent the occurrence of various autonomic disorders. Everyone deserves to enjoy a healthier and happier life every day: this is why everyone needs daily vagus nerve self-stimulation. Vagus nerve self-stimulation is the best way to manage anxiety, stress, and depression. We sincerely hope that by sticking to each exercise provided here, you will enjoy the happier and healthier life you seek.